BLUEPRINTS
Q&A Step 3 Pediatrics

Second Edition

BLUEPRINTS
Q&A Step 3 Pediatrics

Second Edition

Jeffrey L. Foti, MD, FAAP
Attending Pediatrician, Bill Holt Pediatric Infectious Disease Clinic
Phoenix Children's Hospital
Phoenix, Arizona
Clinical Assistant Professor, University of Arizona School of Medicine
Tucson, Arizona

Janice P. Piatt, MD
Medical Director, Bill Holt Pediatric Infectious Disease Clinic
Associate Director, Pediatric Clinic
Phoenix Children's Hospital
Phoenix, Arizona

Series Editor:

Michael S. Clement, MD, FAAP
Mountain Park Health Center
Clinical Lecturer in Family and Community Medicine
University of Arizona College of Medicine
Consultant, Arizona Department of Health Services
Phoenix, Arizona

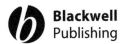
Blackwell
Publishing

© 2005 by Blackwell Publishing

Blackwell Publishing, Inc., 350 Main Street, Malden, Massachusetts 02148-5018, USA
Blackwell Publishing Ltd, 9600 Garsington Road, Oxford OX4 2DQ, UK
Blackwell Publishing Asia Pty Ltd, 550 Swanston Street, Carlton, Victoria 3053, Australia

04 05 06 07 5 4 3 2 1

ISBN: 1-4051-0396-5

Library of Congress Cataloging-in-Publication Data

Blueprints Q&A step 2. Pediatrics / [edited by] Jeffrey L. Foti, Janice P. Piatt.—2nd ed.
    p. ; cm.—(Blueprints. Q&A step 3 series)
    Includes bibliographical references and index.
    ISBN 1-4051-0396-5 (pbk.)
    1. Pediatrics—Examinations, questions, etc.   2. Physicians–Licenses–United States–
Examinations–Study guides.
    [DNLM: 1. Pediatrics—Examination Questions.   WS 18.2 B6582 2005]   I. Title:
Blueprints Q and A step three. Pediatrics.   II. Title: Pediatrics.   III. Foti, Jeffrey L.   IV. Piatt,
Janice P. Series.

    RJ48.2.B582   2005
    618.92′00076—dc22

                                                                                        2004012944
A catalogue record for this title is available from the British Library

Acquisitions: Nancy Anastasi Duffy
Development: Kate Heinle
Production: Debra Murphy
Cover design: Hannus Design Associates
Interior design: Mary McKeon
Typesetter: Techbooks in New Delhi, India
Printed and bound by Capital City Press in Berlin, VT

For further information on Blackwell Publishing, visit our website:
www.blackwellmedstudent.com

Notice: The indications and dosages of all drugs in this book have been recommended in the
medical literature and conform to the practices of the general community. The medications
described do not necessarily have specific approval by the Food and Drug Administration for
use in the diseases and dosages for which they are recommended. The package insert for each
drug should be consulted for use and dosage as approved by the FDA. Because standards for
usage change, it is advisable to keep abreast of revised recommendations, particularly those
concerning new drugs.

The publisher's policy is to use permanent paper from mills that operate a sustainable forestry
policy, and which has been manufactured from pulp processed using acid-free and elementary
chlorine-free practices. Furthermore, the publisher ensures that the text paper and cover board
used have met acceptable environmental accreditation standards.

Contents

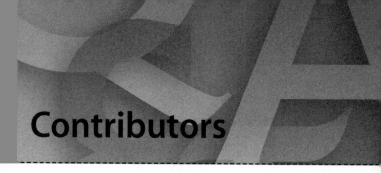

Contributors

Brendan Cassidy, MD
Pediatric Ophthalmologist
Phoenix Children's Hospital
Phoenix, Arizona

Randal C. Christensen, MD, MPH
Clinical Assistant Professor
University of Arizona
Tucson, Arizona
Faculty Physician
Phoenix Children's Hospital
Phoenix, Arizona

Melvin L. Cohen, MD
Director of Medical Education
Phoenix Children's Hospital
Phoenix, Arizona
Clinical Professor, Pediatrics
University of Arizona School of Medicine
Tucson, Arizona

Tala Dajani, MD
Fellow, Pediatric Endocrinology
Phoenix Children's Hospital
Phoenix, Arizona

Joel A. Hahnke, MD
Pediatric Chief Resident
Phoenix Children's Hospital
Phoenix, Arizona

Ronald C. Hansen, MD
Chief, Pediatric Dermatology
Phoenix Children's Hospital
Phoenix, Arizona

John R. Hartley, DO, FAAP
Attending Physician, General Pediatrics
Phoenix Children's Hospital
Phoenix, Arizona

Michelle Huddleston, MD
Clinical Assistant Professor, Pediatrics and Internal Medicine
University of Arizona School of Medicine
Tucson, Arizona
Attending Pediatrician and Clinical Director of
Adolescent Clinic
Phoenix Children's Hospital
Phoenix, Arizona

John Kashani, DO
Banner Good Samaritan Medical Center
Office of Medical Toxicology
Phoenix, Arizona

Frank LoVecchio, DO, MPH
Medical Director
Banner Good Samaritan Poison Control Center
Maricopa Medical Center,
Department of Emergency Medicine
Phoenix, Arizona

Margaret R. Moon, MD, MPH
Director, General Pediatrics Outpatient Clinic
Phoenix Children's Hospital
Phoenix, Arizona

J. Robb Muhm, Jr., MD, MBA
Clinical Assistant Professor
University of Arizona School of Medicine
Tucson, Arizona
General Pediatrician
Phoenix Children's Hospital
Phoenix, Arizona

Kay C. Pinckard-Hansen, MD, FAAP
Faculty, General Pediatrics Department;
Teaching Attending Physician; and
Pediatric Consultant, Rehabilitation Program
Phoenix Children's Hospital
Phoenix, Arizona

Michael Recht, MD, PhD
Director of Hematology
Director, The Hemophilia Center
Division of Hematology/Oncology
Phoenix Children's Hospital
Phoenix, Arizona

Adam J. Schwarz, MD
Clinical Associate Professor, Pediatrics
University of Arizona School of Medicine
Director, Education Program
Division of Pediatric Critical Care
Phoenix Children's Hospital
Phoenix, Arizona

Paul C. Stillwell, MD
Director, Pediatric Pulmonology
Physician in Chief
Phoenix Children's Hospital
Phoenix, Arizona

Jeffrey Weiss, MD
Chief, Section of General Pediatrics
Phoenix Children's Hospital
Phoenix, Arizona
Professor, Clinical Pediatrics
University of Arizona School of Medicine

Mark Yarema, MD FRCPC
Fellow, Department of Medical Toxicology
Banner Good Samaritan Medical Center
Phoenix, Arizona

Reviewers

Nathan Boucher
Class of 2004
Northeastern University Physician Assistant Program
Boston, Massachusetts

Michelle Karen Leggett, MD
PGY-2, Department of Family Practice
David Grant Medical Center
Travis Air Force Base, California

Frederick C. Lewis, MD
Anesthesiology Resident
University of Wisconsin Hospital and Clinics
Madison, Wisconsin

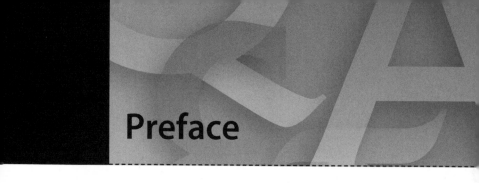

Preface

Thank you! We know that you, our customers, have successfully used the first edition of the Blueprints Q&A series to study for Boards and shelf exams. We also learned that those of you in physician assistant, nurse practitioner, and osteopath programs have found the series helpful to review for Boards and rotation exams.

At Blackwell, we think of our customers as our secret weapon. For every book Blackwell publishes, we rely heavily on the opinions of our customers, and we credit much of our success to the feedback we get from you. Your comments, suggestions—even complaints—help determine everything from content to features to the design of our books. The second edition of the Blueprints Q&A series is an excellent example of how much influence your feedback truly has:

- You asked for more questions per book, so the questions have doubled (200 per book!).
- You wanted questions that better reflect the format of the Boards, so all questions have been updated to match the current USMLE format for Step 3.
- You liked the detailed explanations for every answer—right or wrong—so we made sure that complete correct and incorrect answers were provided for each question.
- You needed a smaller trim size for easier portability, and now you have it. This edition is small enough to fit in a white coat pocket.
- You were looking for an easier way to test yourself, and we redesigned this edition to do just that. Answer keys and tabbed sections make for easier navigation between questions and answers.
- You wanted an index for easy reference and you got it (along with abbreviations and normal lab values).

We hope you like this new edition of the Blueprints Q&A series as much as we do. And keep your suggestions and ideas coming! Please send any comments you may have about this book, or any book in the Blueprints series, to *blue@bos.blackwellpublishing.com*.

The Publisher
Blackwell Publishing

Acknowledgments

Phoenix Children's Hospital, Pediatric Radiology Archives, for supplying a majority of the radiological images used in this book. David Carpientieri, M.D., Pathologist, Phoenix Children's Hospital, for assistance in obtaining and supplying images used in this book. This book is dedicated to Louis and Maria, for your continued love and support.

—*Jeff Foti*

Abbreviations

AAP	American Academy of Pediatrics	CMV	Cytomegalovirus
ABC	Airway, breathing, circulation	CNS	Central nervous system
ABG	Arterial blood gas	CO$_2$	Carbon dioxide/bicarbonate
ACTH	Adrenocorticotropic hormone	CPAP	Continuous positive airway
ADH	Antidiuretic hormone		pressure
ADHD	Attention deficit hyperactivity	CPK	Creatine phosphokinase
	disorder	CPR	Cardiopulmonary resuscitation
AED	Automatic external defibrillator	CRP	C-reactive protein
AFB	Acid fast bacilli	CSF	Cerebrospinal fluid
AFP	Alpha-fetoprotein	CT	Computed tomography
ALL	Acute lymphoblastic leukemia	CXR	Chest radiograph
ALT	Alanine aminotransferase	DDAVP	Vasopressin
AN	Acanthosis nigricans	DDH	Developmental dysplasia of the
ANA	Anti-nuclear antibody		hip
AOM	Acute otitis media	DHEA	Dehydroepiandrosterone
AP	Anterior-posterior	DI	Diabetes insipidus
ARDS	Acute respiratory distress	DIC	Disseminated intravascular
	syndrome		coagulopathy
ASAP	As soon as possible	DKA	Diabetic ketoacidosis
ASD	Atrial septal defect	DM	Diabetes mellitus
ASO	Antistreptolysin O	DMSA	2,3-Dimercaptosuccinic acid
AST	Aspartate aminotransferase	DNA	Deoxyribonucleic acid
AV	Atrioventricular	DTaP	Diphtheria, tetanus, acellular
AZT	Zidovudine		pertussis
BAL	Bronchoalveolar lavage	DTR	Deep tendon reflex
BAL	Dimercaprol	DVT	Deep venous thrombosis
BMP	Basic metabolic panel	EBV	Epstein-Barr virus
BP	Blood pressure	ECG	Electrocardiogram
BPD	Bronchopulmonary dysplasia	ECHO	Echocardiogram
BPM	Beats per minute	ED	Emergency department
BRAT	Banana, rice, applesauce, toast	EDTA	Ethylenediamine tetraacetic acid
BUN	Blood urea nitrogen	EEG	Electroencephalography
C	Celsius	EIA	Exercise-induced asthma
CA	Coronary artery	EKG	Electrocardiogram
CAH	Congenital adrenal hyperplasia	ELISA	Enzyme-linked immunosorbent
CBC	Complete blood count		assay
CDC	Centers for Disease Control	EMG	Electromyography
CF	Cystic fibrosis	ENT	Ear, nose, and throat
CFTR	CF transmembrane regulator	ER	Emergency room
CK	Creatinine kinase	ESR	Erythrocyte sedimentation rate
Cl	Chloride	ETT	Endotracheal tube
CMP	Complete metabolic panel	F	Fahrenheit

FEV	Forced expiratory volume	LUQ	Left upper quadrant
FSGN	Focal segmental glomerulonephritis	LV	Left ventricle
		MCH	Mean corpuscular hemoglobin
FSH	Follicle-stimulating hormone	MCHC	Mean corpuscular hemoglobin concentration
FTT	Failure to thrive		
GBS	Group B streptococcus	MCV	Mean corpuscular volume
GCS	Glasgow Coma Score	MMR	Measles, mumps, rubella
GER	Gastroesophageal reflux	4-MP	Fomepizole
GERD	Gastroesophageal reflux disease	MRA	Magnetic resonance angiography
GH	Growth hormone	MRI	Magnetic resonance imaging
GHB	Gamma hydroxybutyrate	MS	Multiple sclerosis
GI	Gastrointestinal	Na	Sodium
HA	Headache	NaCl	Sodium chloride
HAV	Hepatitis A vaccine	NEC	Necrotizing enterocolitis
Hb	Hemoglobin	NG	Nasogastric
HCG	Human chorionic gonadotropin	NPO	Nothing by mouth
HCO3	Bicarbonate	NPV	Negative predictive value
HEENT	Head, eyes, ears, nose, throat	NS	Normal saline
Hib	Haemophilus influenzae vaccine	NSAID	Nonsteroidal anti-inflammatory drug
HIV	Human immunodeficiency virus		
HPV	Human papilloma virus	OCP	Oral contraceptive pill
HR	Heart rate	OH	Hydroxy
HSP	Henoch-Schönlein purpura	OME	Otitis media with effusion
HSV	Herpes simplex virus	OR	Operating room
HUS	Hemolytic uremic syndrome	OTC	Over the counter
ICP	Intracranial pressure	P	Pulse
IgA	Immunoglobulin A	PCOS	Polycystic ovarian syndrome
IgE	Immunoglobulin E	PCP	Primary care physician
IGF	Insulin growth factor	PCP	Phencyclidine
IGFBP	Insulin-like growth factor binding protein	PCR	Polymerase chain reaction
		PDA	Patent ductus arteriosus
IgG	Immunoglobulin G	PICU	Pediatric intensive care unit
IgM	Immunoglobulin M	PID	Pelvic inflammatory disease
IM	Intramuscular	PO	By mouth
INH	Isoniazid	PPD	Purified protein derivative
IO	Intraosseous	PPV	Positive predictive value
IPV	Inactivated polio	PSGN	Poststreptococcal glomerulonephritis
IQ	Intelligence quotient		
ITP	Idiopathic thrombocytopenic purpura	PT	Prothrombin time
		PTH	Parathyroid hormone
IV	Intravenous	PTT	Partial thromboplastin time
IVF	In vitro fertilization	PTU	Propylthiouracil
IVH	Intraventricular hemorrhage	R	Respirations
IVIG	Intravenous immunoglobulin	RBC	Red blood cell
J	Joule	RDW	Red blood cell distribution width
JRA	Juvenile rheumatoid arthritis		
K	Potassium	RF	Rheumatoid factor
KCl	Potassium chloride	RNA	Ribonucleic acid
Kg	Kilogram	RPR	Rapid plasma reagin
KOH	Potassium hydroxide	RSV	Respiratory syncytial virus
KUB	Kidneys/ureter/bladder radiograph	RV	Right ventricle
		SBE	Subacute bacterial endocarditis
LDH	Lactate dehydrogenase	SCFE	Slipped capital femoral epiphysis
LH	Luteinizing hormone	SCIWORA	Spinal cord injury without radiologic abnormality
LP	Lumbar puncture		

SIADH	Syndrome of inappropriate antidiuretic hormone	TIBC	Total iron binding capacity
SIDS	Sudden infant death syndrome	TM	Tympanic membrane
SLE	Systemic lupus erythematosus	TRH	Thyroid releasing hormone
SMR	Sexual maturity rating	TSH	Thyroid stimulating hormone
SOD	Septo-optic dysplasia	TTN	Transient tachypnea of the newborn
STD	Sexually transmitted disease	UA	Urinalysis
STAT	Immediate	UGI	Upper gastrointestinal tract
SVT	Supraventricular tachycardia	URI	Upper respiratory infection
T	Temperature	UTI	Urinary tract infection
T4	Thyroxine	VSD	Ventricular septal defect
TB	Tuberculosis	VZIG	Varicella-zoster immunoglobulin
Td	Toxoid	WBC	White blood cells
TEF	Tracheoesophageal fistula		

Normal Ranges of Laboratory Values

Blood, Plasma, Serum

Alanine aminotransferase (ALT)	2–40 IU/L
Albumin	3.8–5.4 g/dL
Alkaline phosphatase	42–362 IU/L
Amylase	21–86 IU/L
Anti-nuclear antibody	< 1:40
Antistreptolysin O titer (school-aged child)	170–330 Todd units
Arterial blood gas, child	
pH	7.35–7.45
pCO_2	35–40 mm Hg
pO_2	90–95 mm Hg
HCO_3	22–26 mEq/L
Aspartate aminotransferase (AST)	10–41 IU/L
Bicarbonate	22–28 mEq/L
Bilirubin, total	0.2–1.1 mg/dL
C-reactive protein (CRP)	< 0.3 mg/dL
Calcium	8.8–10.8 mg/dL
CD4 absolute count/% (12 months–6 years)	
No suppression	> 1000/μL/> 25%
Moderate suppression	500–999/μL/15%–24%
Severe suppression	< 500/μL/< 15%
Cerebrospinal fluid, child (CSF)	
WBC	0–7 WBCs/μL
RBC	0 RBCs/μL
Glucose	40–80 mg/dL
Protein	5–40 mg/dL
Chloride	95–105 mEq/L
Cholesterol	< 170 mg/dL
Creatine kinase (CPK)	10–70 U/L
Creatinine	0.6–1.2 mg/dL
Glucose, serum	70–110 mg/dL
HIV viral load	< 50 copies/mL
Lactate dehydrogenase (LDH)	45–90 IU/L
Lead, blood	< 5 μg/dL
Lipase	16–63 IU/L
Magnesium	1.5–2.0 mEq/L
Phosphorus	3.0–4.5 mg/dL
Potassium	3.5–5.0 mEq/L
Protein	5.7–8 g/dL

Rheumatoid factor (RF)	< 1:20
Sodium	136–145 mEq/L
Triglyceride	< 150 mg/dL
Urea nitrogen, blood (BUN)	8–25 mg/dL

Hematologic

Erythrocyte sedimentation rate, child (ESR)	0–10 mm/hr
Hematocrit, child	12.5–16.1 mg/dL
Hemoglobin, child	36%–47%
Leukocyte count and differential	
Leukocyte count	4500–11,000/μL
Segmented neutrophils	54%–62%
Bands	3%–5%
Eosinophils	1%–3%
Basophils	0%–0.75%
Lymphocytes	25%–33%
Monocytes	3%–7%
Mean corpuscular hemoglobin concentration (MCHC)	31–37 g/dL
Mean corpuscular volume (MCV)	75–95 μm^3
Partial thromboplastin time (PTT)	25–40 sec
Platelet count	150,000–400,000/μL
Prothrombin time (PT)	11–15 sec
Red cell distribution width (RDW)	11.5%–14.5%
Reticulocyte count	0.5%–1.5%

Questions

Setting 1: Community-Based Health Center

You work at a community-based health facility where patients seeking both routine and urgent care are encountered. Many patients are members of low-income groups; many are ethnic minorities. Several industrial parks and local businesses send their employees to the health center for treatment of on-the-job injuries and employee health screening. There is a facility that provides X-ray films, but CT and MRI scans must be arranged at other facilities. Laboratory services are available.

1. The left pupil of a 12-month-old girl has been noted to be white by the parents. Recently, she has been rubbing that eye and squinting when exposed to bright light. A full ophthalmic exam is performed, but the retina is poorly visualized even after dilation of the pupil. A massive outpouring of white blood cells is seen in the anterior chamber, and fibrous strands are noted to extend from the iris to the lens consistent with uveitis. The remainder of her physical exam is normal. Which of the following is the most appropriate first step in the management of this patient?

A. CT scan of the orbits
B. The avoidance of steroid eye drops
C. Blood samples for acute and convalescent titers of CMV, toxoplasmosis, syphilis, and toxocara
D. The avoidance of dilating eye drops
E. Titers of anti-nuclear antibody (ANA)

2. A 5-year-old boy is brought into clinic with a history of "white spots on his face" for 2 weeks. The lesions are nonpruritic and appear to have a fine scaly uniform texture (Figure 2). Under Wood's light exam there is no specific fluorescence. The mother thinks they have become worse since the return from his camping trip. Which of the following is the most appropriate management option?

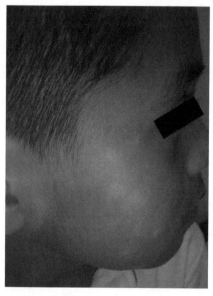

Figure 2 • Image courtesy of the Phoenix Children's Hospital, Phoenix, Arizona.

A. Dermatology referral
B. Griseofulvin
C. Low-potency topical corticosteroid
D. Topical selenium sulfide
E. Diphenhydramine (Benadryl)

3. A 2-year-old boy comes to your clinic for a checkup. He is well except he walks with a slight in-toed gait. When you place him prone on the examination table with his knees flexed and measure the angle formed by the axis of the thigh and the axis of the foot, you note that the foot is internally rotated. You diagnose internal tibial torsion. The best management for this condition at this age is:

    A. Refer to a pediatric orthopedic surgeon for serial casting
    B. Obtain leg radiographs to measure the thigh-foot angle
    C. Suggest high-top, straight last shoes with arch supports
    D. Send patient to be fitted for a Denis-Brown bar
    E. Reassure parents that no treatment is needed at this age

4. You are seeing a 12-year-old girl in clinic because she has ptosis and muscle weakness after repetitive use. You suspect a diagnosis of myasthenia gravis. The best next test to confirm the diagnosis would be:

    A. EMG
    B. EEG
    C. Anti-acetylcholine receptor antibodies assay in the serum
    D. Muscle biopsy
    E. Serum creatine phosphokinase (CPK) level

5. You are seeing a 9-month-old boy for a well-child exam. This is his first visit to the clinic since the age of 2 months because his parents are homeless and have been living in multiple shelters. He has been bottle fed and reportedly began solids around 6 months of age. The mother does not report any excessive spitting-up, feeding problems, or undercurrent illnesses. On exam, he is alert and interactive, but markedly thin. The rest of the physical exam is normal. His growth chart reveals that his head circumference and length have dropped from the 90th to the 75th percentile, while his weight has dropped from the 75th to less than the 25th percentile. CBC, lead level, urinalysis, CMP, thyroid function, HIV, and sweat tests are all normal. The best next step in management would be:

    A. Contrast head MRI
    B. Contrast head CT
    C. Nuclear medicine gastric emptying study
    D. Colonoscopy with biopsies
    E. Hospitalization for observed feedings and calorie count

6. You are seeing a 12-year-old obese female in your clinic for the first time. The mother reports that her baby had a low glucose as a newborn and was very floppy. She had feeding difficulties and grew poorly, requiring nutritional supplements as an infant; she is now overweight. Her mother reports that she is obsessed with food, hides food, and sneaks into the refrigerator at night. She is very behind in school and is in special education classes. On physical exam, she has blue, almond-shaped eyes and blond hair. She has very small hands and feet. Her speech is nasal in quality. She is quite obese, with her weight above the 99th percentile, and is short for her age. Due to your suspicions, you order a chromosomal evaluation. The result shows an abnormality of chromosome 15. Which of the following is accurate counseling about this patient's syndrome?

    A. Hypotonia is progressive, leading to respiratory failure
    B. Mental retardation is uncommon
    C. Ataxia is commonly seen in older children
    D. Obesity and sleep apnea are common in older patients
    E. Cardiac and skeletal defects are common

7. A 6-year-old boy who is in first grade is brought to your clinic because his parents are quite upset about his encopresis. The patient had been successfully toilet trained at 3 years of age, but the mother reports the boy now goes several days without having a bowel movement. His stools are so large in size that there is pain with bowel movements. About three times a week, the patient has loose stool that leaks into his underwear. This is causing great problems with teasing at school. On physical exam, you find a large amount of stool in the rectum. The best next step in the management of this patient is:

A. Institute a low-fiber diet
B. Prescribe enemas or laxatives to evacuate retained stool
C. Have child sit on toilet for at least 30 minutes (or until bowel movement) daily
D. Order a barium enema
E. Refer patient to a child psychiatrist

8. A 3-year-old boy is seen in your clinic because of an apparent ataxia that has been progressive for the past year. Recently he has also developed "bloodshot" eyes, which is not associated with eye drainage. His other significant history shows that he suffers from rather severe and resistant sinopulmonary infections and otitis media. An exam reveals bilateral telangiectasis of the conjunctiva. You are concerned about an immunodeficiency syndrome. Which of the following is the most accurate information to give to the family?

A. This condition is transmitted as an autosomal dominant trait; therefore a parent should have this condition, or it is a result of a genetic mutation
B. Agammaglobulinemia frequently accompanies this condition
C. Thymus hypoplasia is associated with this condition
D. The ataxia which occurs is usually a static condition and not progressive
E. T-cell function is abnormal, and therefore lymphoproliferative disorders are usually of very low incidence

9. A 2-month-old boy is seen at a clinic well-child checkup and is noted to have a head size greater than the 95th percentile. His height and weight are both near the 50th percentile. His head control is poor, and his anterior fontanelle is also quite large. His cranial sutures are slightly separated. A head ultrasound is ordered (Figure 9). Which one of the following statements applies to this patient?

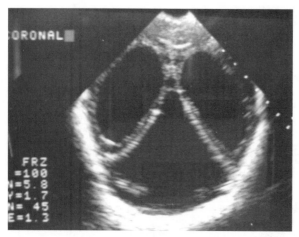

Figure 9 • Image courtesy of the Department of Radiology, Phoenix Children's Hospital, Phoenix, Arizona.

A. The ultrasound exam reveals hydranencephaly
B. The ultrasound is most consistent with a Dandy-Walker cyst
C. A ventricle peritoneal shunt would offer no benefit to this patient
D. This abnormality is generally associated with myelomeningocele
E. This benign condition needs only long-term observation

10. A 3-year-old girl presents with a history of coke-colored urine and periorbital edema. She has previously been well, but was noted to have URI symptoms and a sore throat with fever about 2 weeks ago. These symptoms appeared to resolve spontaneously. Her presumed diagnosis is poststreptococcal glomerulonephritis (PSGN). Which one of the following statements is consistent with this diagnosis?

A. Thinning of the glomerular basement membrane
B. Late development of hypertension
C. Elevated serum antistreptolysin O (ASO) titer, but a negative anti-DNAase titer
D. Decreased renal tubular function
E. A low serum C3 complement

11. You are seeing a term infant in clinic for the first time. The infant was born to a mother who abused cocaine throughout her pregnancy. Which of the following is an associated complication of in utero cocaine exposure that you might expect in this patient?

A. Ventricular septal defect
B. Postterm delivery
C. Hydrocephalus
D. Placenta previa
E. Hearing loss

12. A 6-year-old child is being seen in your clinic for the evaluation of scalp itching. On further exam you notice that the boy's hair reveals evidence of head lice. Which of the following would be appropriate advice for this boy's parents?

A. Head lice are highly contagious as they can jump from person to person
B. Head lice carry contagious diseases
C. Infestation can often occur after sharing clothing or helmets
D. The one-time application of permethrin 1% is inadequate treatment
E. The child should be allowed to return to school once all nits are gone

13. An 8-year-old male is being evaluated in your clinic for obesity. He is in the second grade and has otherwise been healthy and developing appropriately. His body mass index is 32. Which of the following most likely applies to this patient's obesity?

A. His exam is likely to yield normal findings
B. Sleep apnea is an unlikely complication
C. TSH levels are expected to be abnormal
D. A dietary history will be noncontributory
E. The patient is at a decreased risk for slipped capital femoral epiphysis

14. A 2½-year-old male being seen in clinic develops an urticarial rash and facial swelling after tasting peanut butter for the first time. He has had no previous history of urticaria but does have a history of mild atopic dermatitis. Treatment with diphenhydramine improves the symptoms and they gradually clear with continued diphenhydramine administration. The parents are extremely anxious and have a number of questions. Which of the following would be correct information to give to the family?

    A. Peanut allergy will be lifelong
    B. Peanut allergy is more common in adults than in children
    C. Risk factors for peanut allergy include a history of atopy
    D. The prevalence of peanut allergy is decreasing
    E. Peanut allergy is an IgA-mediated phenomenon

15. A 2-month-old with jaundice is seen in your clinic for the first time. The total and direct bilirubin levels are elevated and you are concerned about the possibility of biliary atresia. Which of the following statements about your suspected diagnosis is true?

    A. The condition is usually due to obliteration of the entire extrahepatic biliary tree
    B. Biliary atresia is much more common than neonatal hepatitis
    C. In biliary atresia, an abdominal ultrasound often shows a large gall bladder
    D. A liver biopsy cannot differentiate biliary atresia from neonatal hepatitis
    E. Success of the Kasai procedure is highest if performed after 6 months of life

16. An 18-month-old boy is seen in the clinic for a checkup. You note that he has severe dental decay. The mother is concerned about her son's caries but has heard "many different things about cavities." Which of the following is accurate information to tell this child's mother?

    A. Caries are caused by an overgrowth of *Staphylococcus aureus*
    B. Dental bacterial colonization occurs when a baby is born
    C. The most likely source of bacterial colonization is the mother's oral flora
    D. Children of mothers with high rates of caries are not at greater-than-average risk for developing caries
    E. Dental decay is equally common in rich and poor families

17. A 6-year-old girl is brought to your clinic because of poor weight gain, chronic cough, and intermittent diarrhea. She has a history of asthma and over the last 2 years she has had four bouts of pneumonia that required hospitalization and antibiotic treatment. She takes an inhaled steroid daily, but is on no other medication. What would you do next?

    A. Refer the patient to a nutritionist for a calorie count
    B. Start a leukotriene inhibitor for better asthma control
    C. Obtain a CT scan of the sinuses
    D. Order a sweat chloride test
    E. Refer the patient to a gastroenterologist to rule out Crohn disease

18. A 2-month-old baby comes to your clinic for a checkup. The mother is concerned that the baby has had noisy breathing since shortly after birth. The baby is taking the bottle well and has been gaining weight adequately. On physical exam the baby looks comfortable but has some intermittent inspiratory stridor, which is worsened in the supine position. Which statement about this condition is most accurate?

A. It is a common cause of expiratory wheezing in young infants
B. Symptoms usually appear around 6 months when chest muscles are getting stronger
C. The airway noise is due to collapse of the supraglottic structures during inspiration
D. Even in severe cases of upper airway obstruction, bronchoscopy is not necessary
E. Because symptoms rarely resolve spontaneously, most infants require tracheostomy

19. A 14-year-old girl is seen at your clinic because of significant pain and swelling of her knees and ankles for the past 2 weeks. She has also had intermittent fevers. There is no family history of arthritis. A rheumatoid factor (RF) is negative, an ASO titer is negative, her sedimentation rate is 80, and an ANA is significantly positive. Which one of the following statements is accurate regarding this girl's illness?

    A. There is sufficient evidence in the information given to make the diagnosis of systemic lupus erythematosus (SLE)
    B. The positive ANA has a low sensitivity but a high positive predictive value for the diagnosis of SLE
    C. The presence of a malar rash and a positive anti-DNA antibody test in addition to the findings described will make the diagnosis of SLE
    D. In children and adolescents with SLE, renal disease is uncommon and does not usually contribute to long-term morbidity as it does in adults
    E. Lupus patients usually produce a variety of anti-nuclear antibodies, but it is unusual to find other autoantibodies

20. A 7-year-old boy is referred to you because he is found to have problems concentrating in school. His teacher also notes that his cognition is near the bottom of the class. You take a thorough history and determine that the patient has been exposed to lead in the home. A blood lead level is 30 μg/dL (normal is < 10 μg/dL). The next most appropriate step in managing this patient includes:

    A. Immediate chelation therapy with dimercaprol (BAL) and 2, 3-dimercapto-succinic acid (DMSA)
    B. Removal from the source of exposure
    C. Admission to the hospital for observation and repeat lead levels
    D. Calling child welfare to apprehend the child
    E. Performing x-rays of the long bones

21. A 12-year-old girl is seen in your clinic for a preschool checkup. She is found to have a blood pressure of 135/90. She is at the 75th percentile for height and weight. Her femoral pulses are good. She has no cardiac murmurs. Her examination is normal. A urinalysis is also normal. You confirm the blood pressure readings several times in your clinic, and the blood pressures remain about the same. You also check that the cuff size is normal. You consult the tables for normal blood pressure and find that, for her height and age, the 95th percentile for systolic is 126 and for diastolic is 82. Your next step would be:

    A. Prescribe a mild diuretic
    B. Place her on a low-sodium diet
    C. Obtain a renal ultrasound
    D. Advise her that this blood pressure is at the upper limits of normal for her age
    E. Use a home blood pressure monitor for 24 to 48 hours

22. A 9-year-old boy is seen in your clinic with a skin rash he's had for the past 2 days. The rash is mostly on his trunk, and seems to come and go. The rash is red and slightly raised, appears to migrate, and is nonpruritic. He gives a history of having had a sore throat about 2 weeks ago, and has had some low-grade fevers and joint pains. An ASO titer is 1:625. Which one group of findings would confirm the diagnosis of acute rheumatic fever?

    A. Arthralgia, no fever, and a rash resembling erythema multiforme
    B. Subcutaneous nodules, fever, and arthralgia
    C. Erythema multiforme, arthralgia, and prolonged PR interval
    D. Arthralgia, fever, no rash, and erythrocyte sedimentation rate (ESR) = 120
    E. Arthritis, no fever, and ESR = 10

23. A 13-year-old slender early adolescent girl has been complaining of right hip discomfort for several weeks. An exam reveals significant discomfort when that hip is rotated, and she prefers to keep her hip slightly flexed and externally rotated. Which one of the following is the most accurate information to give to the family?

    A. Endocrine dysfunction need not be considered as causative factor in slipped capital femoral epiphysis
    B. Slipped capital femoral epiphysis occurs most often in obese adolescent girls
    C. About 50% of cases of slipped capital femoral epiphysis in girls occur after puberty
    D. A simple anterior-posterior (AP) pelvis x-ray may not demonstrate a slipped capital femoral epiphysis
    E. Slipped capital femoral epiphysis is not commonly bilateral

24. A 2-year-old boy presents to the clinic and has pallor on exam. His mother states that he drinks 45 ounces of cow's milk a day. A CBC reveals a hemoglobin of 8.2 and a mean corpuscular volume (MCV) of 65. Which of the following indices is compatible with this patient's diagnosis?

    A. Decreased red blood cell distribution width (RDW)
    B. Increased serum ferritin
    C. Increased total iron binding capacity (TIBC)
    D. Increased reticulocyte count
    E. Increased serum iron level

25. A 15-month-old boy is seen in your clinic because of vomiting and diarrhea. He had two episodes of vomiting earlier today, but now he is able to drink small amounts of fluid without emesis. On physical exam, you find the baby to be mildly dehydrated, but the remainder of the exam is completely within normal limits. Rather than hospitalizing the baby for IV fluids, you decide to treat with oral rehydration solution at home. The composition of the oral rehydration solution should be:

    A. 20–30 mEq of sodium per liter; 2% glucose
    B. 40–50 mEq of sodium per liter; no glucose
    C. 50–90 mEq of sodium per liter; no glucose
    D. 50–90 mEq of sodium per liter; 10% to 12% glucose
    E. 50–90 mEq of sodium per liter; 2% glucose

26. A 6-year-old boy is brought to your clinic because of fever and a painful, swollen eye. His mother thinks he may have been bitten by a mosquito on his face yesterday. The inflamed, tense eyelid swelling, which was first noted about 18 hours ago, has progressed so that you are not able to examine the globe adequately. You order a CT scan of the orbit (Figure 26). How will you manage this patient?

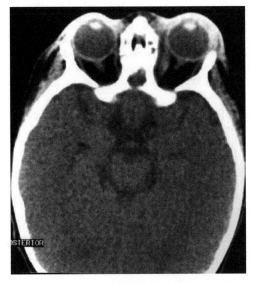

Figure 26 • Image courtesy of Dr. Bangert, Department of Radiology, University Hospitals of Cleveland, Cleveland, Ohio.

A. Admit to the hospital for observation and pain control
B. Administer subcutaneous epinephrine and initiate oral corticosteroids
C. Begin oral administration of amoxicillin and see patient in clinic tomorrow
D. Start oral antihistamine and application of ice directly to the eye every 4 to 6 hours
E. Admit patient to the hospital to start IV antibiotics and obtain surgical consultation

27. A 2-month-old boy is brought to your clinic because of nonbilious, projectile vomiting for 3 days. His parents have noted decreased stool frequency. On physical exam, you see peristaltic gastric waves. Which of the statements about this patient's condition is true?

A. Because of the vomiting, most patients develop metabolic acidosis
B. A palpable, olive-sized mass can sometimes be palpated in the mid-abdomen
C. The presence of jaundice is inconsistent with this condition
D. The diagnosis almost always requires an upper GI series
E. This is a surgical emergency that requires emergent surgery to prevent perforation

28. A 5-month-old African-American baby is brought to your clinic for a checkup. He has been growing well and his physical exam is normal aside from a large umbilical hernia. Which of the following statements about umbilical hernias is true?

A. They usually require surgical repair at some time before the child is 1 year old
B. They are rare in African-American babies
C. Strangulation occurs more often than with inguinal hernias
D. They may be associated with hypothyroidism and mucopolysaccharidoses
E. Taping a coin over the hernia will result in faster resolution

29. A 16-year-old adolescent comes to you concerned and embarrassed about the dark facial hair she is developing. You also note the tendency to excessively dark hair on her arms and legs. On further questioning, she admits to having some on her chest between her breasts and around her nipples. You note that she is obese and is developing dark, velvety, rugated skin on the back of her neck. You are concerned that she may have, or be at risk for, other associated medical problems. Which one of the following is a common misdiagnosis associated with this condition?

- **A.** Poor hygiene and self-care due to her self-consciousness and possible depression
- **B.** Chronic fatty infiltration of the liver and cirrhosis
- **C.** Diabetes mellitus type II
- **D.** Polycystic ovarian syndrome
- **E.** Hypothyroidism

30. A 4-year-old boy has recently moved to your town. At his first well-child visit with you, his mother expresses concern about her child's short stature. His previous growth chart is shown (Figure 30). The patient's father was short as a child, but he is of average adult height. The child is eating and acting well and his development is normal. What is the most appropriate management of this patient?

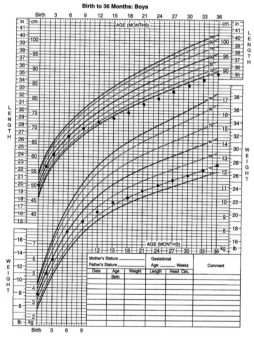

Figure 30 • Image courtesy of the Phoenix Children's Hospital, Phoenix, Arizona. Source: Developed by the National Center for Health Statistics in collaboration with the National Center for Chronic Disease Prevention and Health Promotion (2000). http://www.cdc.gov/growthcharts

- **A.** Referral to an endocrinologist
- **B.** Increase caloric intake and check height again in 3 months
- **C.** Order a CBC, electrolytes, urinalysis, sedimentation rate, and thyroid tests
- **D.** Order radiographs of the hands and wrists to determine the bone age
- **E.** No tests or treatment is needed at this time

31. A 6-month-old boy is brought to your clinic because of URI with rhinorrhea, low-grade fever, and cough. When he cries, the mother says she can hear a high-pitched respiratory sound when he takes a breath in. His cry also sounds hoarse to her. The patient has been able to drink well and appears adequately hydrated. He seems active and happy and is neither tachypneic nor dyspneic. The patient does have a mild barky cough when you examine him. What would be the best next step in the management of this patient?
  A. Order a radiograph of the neck (AP and lateral views)
  B. Prescribe amoxicillin for 10 days
  C. Instruct the parents to use a cool mist vaporizer; encourage oral hydration; no medication needed at this time
  D. Give oral dexamethasone (Decadron); send the patient to the ER for racemic epinephrine treatments
  E. Send the patient to the hospital for admission and airway management

32. A 9-month-old girl is seen in your clinic because her mother reports she is having intermittent abdominal pain associated with vomiting and low-grade fever for the past 24 hours. The baby's stools are noted to contain mucus and blood. On physical exam, you feel a sausage-shaped mass in the right upper quadrant. Which of the following statements about this girl's illness is true?
  A. It is most commonly seen in school-age children
  B. "Currant-jelly" stools (blood and mucus) are seen in almost all cases
  C. The younger the child, the more likely there will be a lead point
  D. Most cases are ileocolic
  E. Barium or air enema will cause reduction in only about 10% to 20% of cases

33. A 1-month-old baby is brought to your clinic for a regular checkup. The exam is completely normal but the mother is concerned that her baby's feet are crooked. The forefoot is deviated medially and there is a prominence at the base of the 5th metatarsal. The forefoot can be easily manipulated into the normal position. In discussing this child's condition with the mother, which is the most accurate information to discuss?
  A. The condition is usually unilateral
  B. Radiologic evaluation should be performed early
  C. Most cases will resolve spontaneously without treatment
  D. Even if the foot is flexible, casting is needed if the foot is not straight by 2 to 3 months
  E. Surgery is required in about half of cases

34. A 12-year-old boy developed sudden onset of grossly bloody urine. He has been a well child, and there have been no serious illnesses in the past. His exam is normal, and he has a normal blood pressure. His urine, indeed, is grossly bloody and there is also 3+ protein. An older brother also has had intermittent gross hematuria. A maternal uncle, age 22, is hard of hearing. Your initial evaluation of this patient would include which one of the following?
  A. Audiogram, examination of the patient's urine, and serum chemistries including blood urea nitrogen (BUN) and creatinine
  B. Reevaluate this patient in 1 month
  C. Schedule for a renal biopsy
  D. Examination of the mother's and uncle's urine
  E. ASO titer

35. A 2-year-old boy is seen with a mild productive cough of 2 weeks' duration. There has been an intermittent low-grade fever, and mild anorexia. There has been no foreign travel, but a grandmother lives in the same house and she has a chronic productive cough. You have some concern that this boy could have tuberculosis (TB). A TB skin test (Mantoux) test is performed, and you decide to get a chest x-ray performed (Figure 35). Which one of the following would apply?

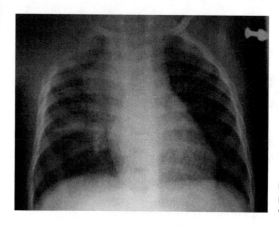

Figure 35 · Image courtesy of the Department of Radiology, Phoenix Children's Hospital, Phoenix, Arizona.

A. Await results of the TB skin test for further action
B. Admit to the hospital for sputum collection for acid fast bacilli (AFB)
C. Start the patient on isoniazid (INH) pending further evaluation
D. Admit to the hospital for nasogastric (NG) aspirate collection for AFB
E. Continued observation and follow-up chest x-ray in 1 month

36. A 12-year-old boy returns home from summer camp. After 2 days he develops frequent watery diarrhea and a mild fever. He is seen in your clinic on the third day of his illness. He looks to be mildly dehydrated and stool examination shows no evidence of blood or white blood cells. His mother is worried that he may have swallowed some water when swimming in the camp lake. The physician discusses the possibilities with the mother and together they decide on a treatment plan. Which of the following would likely be part of that plan?

A. A 3-day trial of erythromycin
B. Admission to the hospital for IV fluids and culture of stool
C. A trial of metronidazole while awaiting giardia antigen
D. Oral rehydration, continued diet, and reevaluation in the next couple of days
E. A call to the local health board requesting investigation of the camp's lake

37. You are seeing a 2-year-old boy in your clinic for evaluation of potential speech delay. The mother states that he has five words and appears to understand all of her commands. After detailed birth history and physical exam with special attention to the head, eyes, ears, nose, and throat (HEENT) exam, you are concerned about a hearing deficit. The best next step in evaluation of a hearing deficit would be:

A. Audiogram
B. Head MRI
C. EEG
D. Speech therapy referral
E. Head CT with special attention to the inner ear structures

38. You are seeing a 6-year-old boy in your clinic for evaluation of headaches. He reports two to three headaches over the past 2 months that are accompanied by the onset of blurry vision followed by severe pounding-type pain. During these headaches his mother states that he lies in a dark room to feel better. You suspect the child is having classic migraines. Which of the following is the best preventative pharmacologic treatment for this child's condition?

A. Sumatriptan (Imitrex)
B. Acetaminophen with codeine
C. Over-the-counter (OTC) analgesia
D. Propranolol
E. There is no effective preventative treatment

39. A 5-year-old boy presents with a history of generalized dependent edema over the past 3 weeks. According to his mother, the patient appears to have gained weight and is using the bathroom less frequently. His exam reveals a distended abdomen with ascites without hepatomegaly, and 3+ pitting edema of the ankles is noted bilaterally. His urinalysis reveals 4+ protein, trace blood, and specific gravity 1.035. Which one of the following is consistent with the diagnosis of minimal change nephrotic syndrome?

A. Low C3 complement level
B. High serum cholesterol and normal triglycerides
C. No immunoglobulin deposition along the glomerular capillary walls
D. Unresponsiveness to glucocorticoid therapy
E. Normal electron microscopy

40. A 4-year-old boy presents to your clinic with fever to 103.4°F and cough. On exam there are crackles present over the left lower lobe region. He has no wheezing. He has been previously healthy. The chest radiograph shows a consolidative infiltrate in the left lower lobe behind the heart, consistent with pneumonia. Which of the following statements about this patient is most likely to be correct?

A. The most likely bacterial etiology is *Streptococcus pneumoniae*
B. The most likely infectious etiology is respiratory syncytial virus (RSV)
C. This cannot be *Mycobacterium tuberculosis* because the pneumonia is in a lower lobe
D. This is characteristic of foreign body aspiration
E. This patient will likely develop a pleural effusion

41. You are seeing an 8-month-old child with an undescended testis in your clinic. This patient is managed most appropriately with:
   A. Monitoring only; testis is likely to descend within the next 6 months
   B. Trial of hormone therapy if no descent by 12 months
   C. Ultrasound evaluation to identify an intra-abdominal testis
   D. Referral to a urologist for further management
   E. MRI evaluation to identify an intra-abdominal testis

42. You are seeing a newborn infant in clinic for the first time. The infant's first-time parents are anxious and concerned about the baby's movements and are worried that something is wrong. Which of the following reflexes is normally absent in a newborn?
   A. Startle (Moro)
   B. Hand grasp
   C. Crossed adductor
   D. Toe grasp
   E. Protective equilibrium

43. A 6-year-old boy is seen in your clinic for a 4-cm oval polymorphic macular rash located over the lower mid-abdominal skin. The most likely diagnosis is:
   A. Scabies
   B. Henoch-Schönlein purpura (HSP)
   C. Poison ivy
   D. Nickel dermatitis
   E. Psoriasis

44. A 4-year-old girl is brought to your clinic with the complaint of persistent rhinorrhea for the past 2 months. Her mother also notes red itchy eyes. On physical exam, you find that the patient is mouth breathing and has dark circles under the eyes. There is a watery nasal discharge and edematous, boggy, bluish mucous membranes with no erythema. Which of the following statements about this condition is most accurate?
   A. Children whose mothers smoke heavily are not at greater risk for allergic rhinitis
   B. A horizontal skinfold over the bridge of the nose is sometimes seen
   C. Neutrophils are seen on a nasal smear
   D. It is okay for dogs and cats to remain in the home
   E. Oral antihistamines and intranasal corticosteroids are generally ineffective

45. A 4-year-old girl presents with a chief complaint of hair loss. On exam, she has a 5-cm area of alopecia on the scalp over her left ear. This is also seen to a lesser degree on the right side of her head. Closer examination of the skin of the scalp in these areas reveals smooth and shiny skin, with no evidence of tiny broken hairs or irritation of the underlying scalp. What is this patient's most likely diagnosis?
   A. Tinea capitus
   B. Traction alopecia
   C. Trichotillomania
   D. Alopecia areata
   E. Contact dermatitis to a hair product

46. A 1-month-old boy presents to your clinic with feeding intolerance, poor weight gain, and a large tongue. On exam, you notice a large posterior fontanelle and umbilical hernia. Your next step in making the diagnosis would be:

A. Abdominal radiograph
B. CBC and blood culture
C. Barium swallow
D. Follow-up on newborn screen results
E. Admit to the hospital for failure-to-thrive (FTT) work-up

47. An otherwise healthy girl comes to your clinic for evaluation of a bright red facial rash and a lacy, reticulated rash on her chest (Figure 47). The girl has been acting and eating normally. She is afebrile and non-toxic appearing. The best management for this situation is:

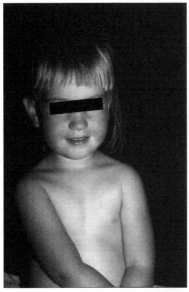

Figure 47 · Image courtesy of the Phoenix Children's Hospital, Phoenix, Arizona.

A. Give the patient amoxicillin for 5 days
B. Keep the patient home from school for 1 week
C. Hospitalize the patient and administer IV gammaglobulin
D. Give all of the patient's classmates parvovirus vaccine
E. The patient needs no treatment; her classmates need no postexposure prophylaxis

48. A 16-year-old female is seen in your clinic with a complaint of irregular periods. She started menstruating at age 12 but has only intermittent periods, about every 3 to 4 months, some very heavy and some very light. Her mother is concerned that she may be pregnant. Her physical exam is significant for obesity, mildly increased facial hair, and pigmentation behind her neck at the hairline and in the axilla. Which of the following lab values would help you confirm the diagnosis?

    A. Elevated TSH
    B. Low testosterone levels
    C. Decreased LH/FSH ratio
    D. Elevated serum dehydroepiandrosterone sulfate (DHEA-S)
    E. Normal lipid profile

The next 2 questions (items 49–50) correspond to the following vignette.

A 13-year-old female complains of heavy menses. Menarche occurred 3 months ago. Her periods are irregular and consist of bleeding for 5 to 7 days. She denies passing any blood clots. She has to change her pad once during the night and 4 to 5 times during the day. There are no bleeding disorders in her family. Her hemoglobin is 10.

49. What is the most likely etiology of her menometrorrhagia?

    A. Pregnancy
    B. Idiopathic thrombocytopenic purpura (ITP)
    C. Cervical polyp
    D. Foreign body
    E. Immature hypothalamic-pituitary-ovarian axis

50. Which of the following would be the most appropriate management of the patient above with dysfunctional bleeding?

    A. Observe
    B. Start iron therapy
    C. Initiate oral contraceptives
    D. Ibuprofen during menses
    E. Transfuse with 15 cc/kg of packed red blood cells
    F. Start iron therapy and initiate oral contraceptives
    G. Start iron therapy, initiate oral contraceptives, and administer ibuprofen during menses
    H. Transfuse with 15 cc/kg of packed red blood cells, and administer ibuprofen during menses

End of set

Answers and Explanations

ONE

Answer Key

1. A	18. C	35. D
2. C	19. C	36. D
3. E	20. B	37. A
4. A	21. E	38. D
5. E	22. B	39. C
6. D	23. D	40. A
7. B	24. C	41. D
8. C	25. E	42. E
9. B	26. E	43. D
10. E	27. B	44. B
11. A	28. D	45. D
12. D	29. A	46. D
13. A	30. E	47. E
14. C	31. C	48. D
15. A	32. D	49. E
16. C	33. C	50. G
17. D	34. A	

1. **A.** One of the more dangerous conditions that may present as leukocoria in this age group is retinoblastoma. Retinoblastoma should be ruled out before an extensive further work-up is initiated, particularly in the otherwise asymptomatic child. In addition to a full eye exam, radiographic evaluation of the globe for calcification is critical. Because an MRI may miss the calcification, a CT scan is considered the imaging study of choice.

B. With careful monitoring by an ophthalmologist, aggressive steroid use is the key to reducing this uveitis.

C. The more common infectious, or peri-infectious causes of leukocoria include CMV, toxoplasmosis, syphilis, and toxocara. These entities should be considered *after* retinoblastoma has been ruled out. Tuberculosis and rubella can also create this form of inflammation. There are hundreds of other infectious agents that can be underlying the uveitis, but clinical suspicion must guide evaluation.

D. In order to prevent papillary occlusion with 360° scarring of the iris border to the lens, dilation of the pupillary sphincter is performed. The strength and frequency of the agent used depends on the degree of inflammation and presence of iris adhesions.

E. This particular patient has no other symptoms of fever, arthritis, or rash to suggest the initial diagnosis of juvenile rheumatoid arthritis (JRA). Although JRA is unusual at this age, it certainly occurs, and must be considered in the evaluation *after* retinoblastoma has been ruled out. Pauciarticular, rheumatoid factor (RF)-negative, ANA-positive patients need to be screened about every 3 months because their uveitis can have such an insidious onset.

2. **C.** The patient in this picture has pityriasis alba, a common skin disorder that presents with discrete areas of hypopigmentation typically on the face, neck, and upper trunk. The underlying etiology is unknown but the lesions appear or are often worsened by sun exposure. Topical corticosteroids and lubrication have been shown to help with resolution of the lesions.

A. There is no need for dermatology referral at this point, although vitiligo should be considered in the differential diagnosis.

B. Griseofulvin would be indicated for the treatment of tinea corporis.

D. Topical selenium sulfide shampoo would be useful for the treatment of tinea versicolor, another entity to consider in the differential. Tinea versicolor is typically more widespread on the trunk, upper extremities, and occasionally on the face; the lesions are also more prominent following sun exposure. They would be expected to have a copper-orange or bronzed appearance under Wood's light.

E. Diphenhydramine (Benadryl) would be indicated to control pruritis.

3. **E.** Reassure the parents that internal tibial torsion is a common condition that causes an in-toed gait.

A, C, D. The condition resolves spontaneously and requires no casts, special shoes, bars, or braces.

B. Radiographs are not necessary. As in this case, the diagnosis is made from the physical exam.

4.   **A.** The EMG results in myasthenia gravis are more specific than a muscle biopsy. The muscle potentials would be expected to fall quickly in amplitude with repetitive stimulation.

   B. An EEG will not reveal any information regarding muscle function.

   C. Anti-acetylcholine antibodies are not always demonstrated in the serum.

   D. Muscle biopsies are generally not helpful in patients with myasthenia gravis.

   E. CPK level should be normal in patients with myasthenia gravis.

5.   **E.** Nonorganic failure to thrive, as suspected in this scenario, can both be diagnosed and treated with observed feedings and a calorie count within a supervised inpatient setting.

   A, B, C, D. Any further radiographic or invasive diagnostic procedures should be reserved until it is firmly established that the child does not gain weight on adequate calories.

6.   **D.** This patient has Prader-Willi syndrome, which is associated with interstitial deletion of chromosome 15. Typical features include severe hypoglycemia and hypotonia in the newborn period. Infants usually have feeding difficulties and grow poorly. Older children commonly develop an excessive appetite and can become morbidly obese, which further contributes to sleep apnea.

   A. The hypotonia can be very severe in infancy but usually abates between 6 months and 6 years.

   B. Mental retardation is seen in virtually all patients with Prader-Willi syndrome. Retardation is mild in 63%, moderate in 31%, and severe in 6%.

   C. Ataxia is not a feature of Prader-Willi syndrome.

   E. Cardiac and skeletal defects are not part of Prader-Willi syndrome.

7.   **B.** Encopresis (passage of feces into inappropriate places) is a complication of chronic constipation. In encopresis, loose stool usually leaks out around the large, hard, retained stool in the rectum. The most important initial step in the treatment of chronic constipation is complete evacuation of any retained stool in the rectum. As long as the rectum is dilated, rectal tone will remain low and regular stooling will not be achieved. Use of hypertonic phosphate enemas is usually tried first. If enemas are unsuccessful, NG administration of hypertonic electrolyte solutions with polyethylene glycol may be needed. Patients with chronic constipation will also need therapy to prevent reaccumulation of stool. This is often done with lubricants (mineral oil) or mild laxatives (senna). High-fiber diets are recommended. Bowel training and behavioral therapy are also very important.

   A. As in the explanation for B, high-fiber diet is recommended.

   C. On a daily basis, on awakening and after dinner, the child should sit on the toilet and attempt to have a bowel movement. However, an excessive amount of time, such as 30 minutes, spent on the toilet can have a negative effect.

D. Most patients with chronic constipation and encopresis will not require a barium enema. However, a history of delayed passage of meconium/stool in the first 48 hours or chronic constipation since birth would be suspicious for Hirschsprung disease and mandate further investigation with a barium enema and subsequent rectal biopsy.

E. Patients who do not respond to medical treatment or who have obvious emotional stressors may benefit from seeing a child psychiatrist. Biofeedback techniques have also been helpful in many cases. The prognosis is usually good and many patients are better in 4 to 6 months.

8. **C.** This patient's syndrome is ataxia-telangiectasia (Louis-Bar syndrome). Thymic hypoplasia with poor organization and lack of Hassall corpuscles is a common feature.

A. Ataxia-telangiectasia is transmitted as an autosomal recessive trait. The abnormal gene is located on chromosome 11, and the gene product is a DNA-dependent protein kinase involved in mitogenic signal transduction.

B. Gammaglobulin abnormalities are associated with ataxia-telangiectasia, but agammaglobulinemia is not present. IgG is usually low, and IgA is frequently absent. IgM may be of low molecular weight.

D. The ataxia in ataxia-telangiectasia is progressive, and these patients are usually confined to a wheelchair in middle or late childhood.

E. In ataxia-telangiectasia, CD3 and CD4 T-cells are moderately reduced. These patients are at increased risk of lymphoreticular cancers, and even adenocarcinomas.

9. **B.** This ultrasound reveals a large fluid-filled cyst in the posterior fossa, with proximal dilatation of the ventricular system. A Dandy-Walker cyst results from developmental failure of the roof of the fourth ventricle during embryogenesis. The resulting dilatation of the fourth ventricle results in a cystic appearance, and most of these infants develop hydrocephalus and progressive neurological impairment. Shunting procedures will help reduce the neurological sequelae.

A. In hydranencephaly there are only remnants of the cerebrum and cerebral cortex, and the remainder of the cranium is filled with fluid.

C. A shunting procedure would relieve the increasing hydrocephalus and allay much of the neurological impairment in Dandy-Walker malformation.

D. The hydrocephalus related to myelomeningocele is generally associated with elongation of the fourth ventricle and kinking of the brain stem, with displacement of the pons and medulla into the cervical canal. The fourth ventricle is not usually cystic. Shunting procedures are used to allay the effects of increasing hydrocephalus.

E. Most Dandy-Walker malformations are not benign and will require shunting.

10. **E.** While the C3 can be normal, it is low in about 90% of cases. This is the only listed feature which would be expected.

A. Endocapillary proliferation of mesangial cells and polymorphonuclear infiltration in the glomeruli are characteristic pathologic findings in PSGN. Basement membranes are not thin in this disease.

B. Hypertension is expected, most often secondary to fluid retention, and occurs early.

C. The immunologic response to streptococcal antigens is usually seen early in PSGN, but is not limited to ASO. Other anti-strep titers such as anti-streptokinase, anti-DNAase, and anti-NADase are also elevated.

D. Tubular function is often spared. Glomerular filtration is impaired secondary to the proliferative process and immune complex deposition that occurs in the glomeruli.

11. **A.** In utero exposure to cocaine has been associated with a number of complications that include cardiac defects, intracranial hemorrhage, necrotizing enterocolitis, placental abruption, as well as low apgars, prematurity, fetal distress, intrauterine growth retardation, and genitourinary malformations. Long-term sequelae include behavioral problems, attention and concentration deficits, and an increased probability of learning disabilities.

B. Preterm, rather than postterm, delivery is associated with intrauterine cocaine exposure.

C. Microcephalus, rather than hydrocephalus, is associated with intrauterine cocaine exposure.

D. Placental abruption, rather than placenta previa, is associated with intrauterine cocaine exposure.

E. Hearing loss has not specifically been shown to be related to cocaine exposure.

12. **D.** Following the one-time treatment of permethrin 1% rinse for head lice, it is suspected that about 20% to 30% of the eggs will still remain. For this reason it is recommended that retreatment occur approximately 7 to 10 days later.

A. Head lice are transmitted usually by direct contact with an infected human source. They cannot fly or jump as commonly thought.

B. Head lice themselves do not carry infectious diseases. Secondary staphylococcal or streptococcal infections may occur following excessive scalp itching.

C. Head lice require a human host to survive. Without a host, they typically die within 1 day. The theoretic risk of transmission from inanimate objects is therefore thought to be extremely rare.

E. The American Academy of Pediatrics (AAP) recommends that a healthy child should not be excluded from school for head lice. Much controversy exists over "no nit" policies and it is believed that by the time the diagnosis of head lice has been made, more than a month of infestation has probably been ongoing.

13. **A.** Obesity is becoming more of a problem in the younger pediatric population. In a majority of cases, a thorough dietary history of increased caloric intake, coupled with the lack of physical activity and positive family history of obesity, will be essential in arriving at the diagnosis. The physical exam will be normal in most cases as will laboratory testing.

B, E. Obesity increases the risk factor for further development of insulin resistance and hence diabetes, as well as complications of hyperlipidemia, sleep apnea, slipped capital femoral epiphysis, and a variety of other disorders.

C. Although screening for hypothyroidism in circumstances of excessive weight gain is certainly reasonable, there are no other symptoms such as dry hair, hypothermia, or bradycardia to suggest this diagnosis.

D. As in the explanation for A, a dietary history of excessive caloric intake would be expected in this child. Further dietary modifications and possible consultation with a nutritionist would be essential in the management of an obese child.

14. **C.** Risk factors for peanut allergy include family history, atopy, maternal exposure to peanuts in the diet, soymilk exposure, and peanut oil exposure to the skin. It would be useful to educate the family regarding future potential exposures and have them educated in first aid and CPR. In case of emergencies, a prescription for an Epipen Jr and instructions on its use is essential.

A. Up to 25% of children will outgrow peanut allergy.

B. Peanut allergy is one of the most common types of food allergy in children.

D. The prevalence of peanut allergy is actually increasing.

E. Peanut allergy is mediated by IgE.

15. **A.** While biliary atresia can occasionally be due to intrahepatic obstruction, 85% of cases are due to obliteration of the extrahepatic ducts.

B. Biliary atresia is seen in 1 in 10,000 to 15,000 births, while neonatal hepatitis is found in 1 in 5000 to 10,000 births.

C. The gall bladder may be small or absent in bilary atresia, but the same ultrasound findings can be seen with neonatal hepatitis, cystic fibrosis, or total parenteral nutrition.

D. A percutaneous liver biopsy is the best test to differentiate biliary atresia from neonatal hepatitis. Biliary atresia is characterized by bile duct proliferation, bile plugs, portal edema, or fibrosis, with the basic hepatic lobular architecture remaining intact. By contrast, in neonatal hepatitis there is severe hepatocellular disease with inflammatory cells and focal necrosis, but with little change in the bile ductules.

E. It is important to consider the diagnosis of biliary atresia early in any child with direct hyperbilirubinemia; the success of the Kasai procedure is highest if performed in the first 8 weeks of life. Delay in diagnosis and surgical management of cholestasis will lead to progressive bile duct obliteration and cirrhosis.

16. **C.** The most common source of dental flora is the mother or another intimate care provider. Caries should be considered an infectious and preventable disease that is vertically transmitted from mothers or other intimate caregivers to infants. Prevention of maternal dental decay will decrease the likelihood of caries in the baby.

A. Dental caries results from an overgrowth of normal bacterial flora (*Streptococcus mutans*, Lactobacillus).

B. Babies become colonized between 6 and 30 months of life.

D. The mother's dental history has a direct correlation on the development of caries in the baby. If the mother has frequent sugar intake, low fluoride exposure, poor oral hygiene, active decay or multiple fillings, and/or infrequent dental visits, the baby is more likely to have caries. Dental flora can be inhibited and caries prevented by fluoride intake, good hygiene, and avoidance of sugary foods. Children who sleep with bottles or breastfeed throughout the night are more likely to get dental decay.

E. Low socioeconomic status has also been identified as a risk factor for caries.

17. **D.** A child with poor weight gain, diarrhea, and multiple bouts of wheezing and pneumonia should be evaluated for cystic fibrosis (CF) with a sweat chloride test. CF is an autosomal recessive transmitted disease caused by a mutation of the CF transmembrane regulator (CFTR) gene on chromosome 7. Typical clinical findings in CF include acute or persistent respiratory symptoms, failure to thrive with malnutrition, malabsorption and/or abnormal stools, rectal prolapse, nasal polyps, sinus disease, and chronic liver disease.

A. Inadequate caloric intake is rarely a cause of poor growth in a child of this age.

B. The diagnosis of asthma may be incorrect in this case, especially given the history of poor weight gain. Patients with CF will often wheeze and present as uncontrolled asthmatics.

C. Sinusitis has been shown to cause wheezing and patients with CF often get sinusitis. In this case, however, there are no signs or symptoms of sinusitis, except for chronic cough.

E. CF is associated with malabsorption due to pancreatic insufficiency. The strong respiratory history is more typical of CF than of Crohn disease.

18. **C.** The noisy breathing in cases of laryngomalacia results from soft airway cartilage and the resultant collapse of supraglottic structures during inspiration.

A. Laryngomalacia is the most common congenital laryngeal abnormality and the most frequent cause of stridor in infants. Laryngomalacia does not cause expiratory wheezing.

B. The symptoms appear within 2 weeks of life and increase in severity for up to 6 months.

D. Because some cases are associated with other airway structural abnormalities, bronchoscopy may be indicated in more severe cases. A patient with swallowing dysfunction will require a contrast swallow study and esophagram. Among other conditions that must be considered in an infant with stridor are congenital and acquired subglottic stenosis, papillomas, vocal cord paralysis, and congenital laryngeal webs and atresia.

E. In most cases, the stridor disappears as the child becomes older. Tracheostomy is rarely needed.

19. **C.** A malar rash and a positive anti-DNA antibody test (immunologic disorder) are both diagnostic criteria for lupus. The arthritis and positive ANA that this patient has are two more criteria. Therefore, this patient has the necessary four of the 11 criteria to make the diagnosis of SLE. The other seven criteria are discoid rash, photosensitivity rash, oral ulcers, serositis, nephritis, neurologic disease, and hematologic disorder.

A. This patient has arthritis and a positive ANA, both major criteria in the diagnosis of lupus. However, four of 11 criteria are needed to confirm the diagnosis and this patient is exhibiting only two.

B. In addition to lupus, a positive ANA can occur with certain drugs, JRA, other collagen vascular diseases, infectious mononucleosis, chronic active hepatitis, and normal individuals. The absence of ANA in childhood lupus is rare. Therefore, an ANA has high sensitivity (percentage with disease who will test positive) and a low positive predictive value (percentage of those with a positive test who will have the disease).

D. Lupus nephritis in children and adolescents is a major cause of long-term morbidity, and frequently culminates in chronic renal failure.

E. Lupus patients have a very active immune system and frequently produce a variety of autoantibodies such as anti-phospholipid, anti-thyroid, anti-coagulant, and Coombs antibodies. Such antibodies are responsible for some of the protean manifestations in lupus patients.

20. **B.** Aggressive environmental intervention is important for lead levels between 25 and 45 µg/dL. With a blood lead level of 30 µg/dL, the first step would be to have the local public health authorities perform a home visit to determine the risk factors within the home and to take steps to remove the child from exposure. At this lead level, environmental intervention to remove lead from the home is the most appropriate approach.

A. Chelation therapy is recommended for lead levels between 45 and 70 µg/dL.

C. Admission to the hospital for observation and repeat lead levels is not necessary unless chelation is planned.

D. A referral to public health authorities, rather than child welfare services, is more appropriate in this setting.

E. X-rays of the long bones can show dense bands at the metaphyses that occur after months to years of exposure. However, normal x-rays do not rule out lead exposure. The most important approach to managing this patient is eliminating the source of lead.

21. **E.** Studies have shown that ambulatory blood pressure monitoring can identify significant hypertension much better than intermittent measurements. It is the best way to rule out "white coat" hypertension.

A. Any treatment for high blood pressure is not appropriate until significant hypertension is confirmed. Significant hypertension is defined as BP readings consistently above the 95th percentile for height and age.

B. Sodium restriction would be recommended if the blood pressure was confirmed to be in the hypertensive range.

C. A renal ultrasound would be useful once significant hypertension has been confirmed by ambulatory monitoring.

D. Advising that this blood pressure is in the upper normal range for her age would suggest you do not know the definition of hypertension.

22. **B.** Using Jones criteria, subcutaneous nodules are a major criterion, and fever and arthralgia are minor criteria. One major, two minors, and evidence of recent group A streptococcal infection makes the diagnosis. The major Jones criteria include migratory polyarthritis, carditis, subcutaneous nodules, erythema marginatum, and Sydenham chorea. The minor criteria include fever, arthralgia, elevated ESR/C-reactive protein (ESR/CRP), and prolonged PR interval.

A. Arthralgia is a minor criterion and erythema marginatum is a major criterion. Required are two majors, or one major and two minors, plus evidence of a preceding group A streptococcus infection. There is not enough evidence for the diagnosis.

C. Using Jones criteria, there is no major manifestation of rheumatic fever here. Arthralgia and prolonged PR interval are minor manifestations, and erythema multiforme is neither a major nor a minor manifestation. See explanation for A for the full diagnostic criteria.

D. Arthralgia, fever, and elevated ESR/CRP are three minor criteria. See explanation for A for the full diagnostic criteria.

E. Arthritis is a major criterion, but there are no minor manifestations. Even though there is evidence of a recent group A streptococcus infection, there is not enough evidence for the diagnosis.

23. **D.** In early slipped capital femoral epiphysis (SCFE) the AP radiograph may not demonstrate the abnormality. A frog lateral is the best x-ray view and should be obtained in all suspected cases of SCFE.

A. SCFE can be seen as a complication of an underlying endocrine disease, such as hypothyroidism. When SCFE occurs before puberty, an investigation for a systemic disease or endocrine disorder is warranted.

B. SCFE occurs more commonly in obese adolescent patients with a 3:1 male predominance, but it does occur also in tall thin adolescents with a recent growth spurt and delayed skeletal maturation.

C. SCFE is not commonly seen in females beyond puberty.

E. Patients with SCFE have a 30% incidence of occurrence on the other side.

24. **C.** The patient suffers from iron deficiency anemia secondary to microscopic GI blood loss from excessive milk ingestion; 18 to 20 ounces of milk per day would be more appropriate. The total iron binding capacity is increased with iron deficiency anemia as iron binding sites are more available.

A. The RDW measures variations in the size of RBCs and increases with iron deficiency.

B. Serum ferritin levels decline and are the earliest marker of iron deficiency. Serum ferritin is also an acute phase reactant that can become elevated in the presence of inflammation.

D. The reticulocyte count measures circulating immature RBCs and decreases with iron deficiency.

E. Decreased serum iron levels would be expected as iron stores in the bone marrow are depleted.

25. **E.** Many babies who are not seriously dehydrated can be treated with oral solutions, thus avoiding hospitalization and complications of IV fluid therapy. Rehydration fluids should contain a high sodium content (50–90 mEq/L) and a small amount of glucose (2.0% to 2.5%). Oral rehydration uses a process called cotransport, in which a molecule of glucose promotes the absorption of a molecule of sodium from the small intestine. As sodium is rapidly absorbed from the intestine, water absorption follows.

A. This solution does not contain enough sodium to promote adequate water absorption from the gut lumen.

B, C. A small amount of glucose is needed for the cotransport process.

D. Solutions high in glucose have a high osmotic load and will draw water into the lumen of the intestine, rather than promoting sodium and water absorption, potentially worsening the diarrhea. Juices, soft drinks, and punches are not appropriate for oral rehydration because they lack sodium and have a high glucose content.

26. **E.** The CT scan of the orbit demonstrates the presence of purulent material in the orbit, typical of orbital cellulitis. Orbital cellulitis may be associated with decreased or painful ocular movement, proptosis (protrusion of eye), or chemosis (edema of the bulbar conjunctiva due to poor venous or lymphatic drainage). Commonly, the lids are so swollen that an adequate examination is impossible and a CT scan is needed to evaluate the orbital contents. Infection often is secondary to sinusitis. Empiric antibiotic coverage should provide activity against *S. aureus, Streptococcus pyogenes, S. pneumoniae, H. influenza, M. catarrhalis,* and anaerobic bacteria of the upper respiratory tract. Ampicillin-sulbactam would be a good choice. If there is a large, well-defined abscess, complete ophthalmoplegia, or vision impairment, surgical drainage of the abscess and the adjacent sinus may be necessary.

A. Orbital cellulitis is a dangerous condition that requires immediate IV antibiotic administration and surgical evaluation.

B. A swollen eye due to an allergic reaction from a mosquito bite is not usually painful and tense. The CT scan would show periorbital swelling, but the orbit would appear normal. Periorbital (preseptal) cellulitis may also cause a swollen eye with a normal orbital scan. This condition requires antibiotic administration, but does not generally need surgical consultation.

C. Amoxicillin would not provide adequate treatment for the organisms that commonly cause orbital cellulitis.

D. Antihistamines and local application of ice are not appropriate treatments for this child.

27. **B.** In cases of pyloric stenosis, there may be a palpable, hard, mobile, nontender mass in the epigastrium, just to the right of the midline. Visible peristaltic waves may be seen, especially just after the baby has been fed.

A. With persistent vomiting there is loss of potassium as well as hydrogen ion and chloride, resulting in the classic presentation of a hypokalemic, hypochloremic metabolic alkalosis.

C. Jaundice can been seen with pyloric stenosis and other forms of intestinal obstruction.

D. When accompanied by the typical history of projectile vomiting after feeding, the presence of the two physical findings of peristaltic gastric waves and a palpable olive-sized mass makes further diagnostic studies unnecessary.

E. Pyloric stenosis is a medical emergency, not a surgical emergency. Bowel necrosis and perforation are not complications of pyloric stenosis. Electrolyte abnormalities should be corrected prior to surgery.

28. **D.** Umbilical hernias are often seen in low-birth weight babies and in babies with certain metabolic abnormalities, such as hypothyroidism and mucopolysaccharidoses.

A. Umbilical hernias usually resolve spontaneously. Because strangulation is extremely rare, surgical correction is not usually recommended unless the hernia persists past age 4 or 5 years or if the abdominal wall defect is very large (greater than 2 cm).

B. Umbilical hernias are much more common in African-American babies.

C. Strangulation of umbilical hernias is rare and much less common than with inguinal hernias.

E. Taping a coin over the abdominal wall defect in order to keep the hernia from protruding is not effective and may actually delay spontaneous closure.

29. **A.** The dark, velvety, rugated skin on the back of her neck is acanthosis nigricans (AN) and is not due to poor hygiene as is sometimes misdiagnosed.

B, C, D, E. Although AN is most commonly associated with type II diabetes mellitus, it can be associated with all of the other disorders listed as well: chronic fatty infiltration of the liver and cirrhosis, polycystic ovarian syndrome, and hypothyroidism.

30.   **E.** This child's growth pattern is typical of constitutional growth delay. The birth height is normal, the child's height velocity drops off at about 1 year of age, and the child is growing at a normal rate again by 3 years of age. Commonly, the parent of the same gender had short stature as a child but attained normal height as an adult. The growth pattern and family history in this case are typical of constitutional growth delay; no further tests are needed. Of course, if normal growth had not resumed by 3 years of age, further evaluation would have been needed.

A. Referral to an endocrinologist is expensive and unnecessary.

B. The child is eating an adequate diet. Excessive caloric intake could cause obesity.

C. These tests would be valuable in the determining the cause of short stature due to an organic disease. This child's growth pattern should be considered a normal variant.

D. The bone age in patients with constitutional growth delay will be less than their chronological age. The discrepancy between bone age and chronological age can be used to counsel parents that their child has the potential for catch-up growth. Typically, when other children stop growing in late adolescence, teens with constitutional growth delay continue to grow and catch up to their peers.

31.   **C.** In this case, the history and physical exam are very typical of viral croup (laryngotracheobronchitis). Croup occurs primarily in the fall and winter and is most often caused by parainfluenza and respiratory syncytial viruses. Patients usually have signs and symptoms of upper respiratory tract infection, a characteristic barky cough, and inspiratory stridor. Viral croup is common in children under age 3. Most children with viral croup can be managed as outpatients with supportive care, oral hydration, humidified air, and parental reassurance.

A. The typical radiographic finding in croup is subglottic edema with the classic "steeple sign"; however, most patients do not need radiographic studies unless there is concern about epiglottitis, foreign body aspiration, or other causes of sever upper airway obstruction.

B. Because croup is a viral illness, antibiotics are not necessary.

D. In moderately severe cases, hospitalization can sometimes be avoided by the use of racemic epinephrine inhalation treatments and a single dose of dexamethasone given via the IM, IV, or oral route.

E. The most severe cases of croup should be hospitalized and may even require endotracheal intubation and management in a pediatric intensive care unit. As the patient in this scenario is well hydrated without any signs of respiratory distress, hypoxia, or resting stridor, outpatient management is more appropriate at this time.

32.   **D.** An intussusception is the telescoping of a part of the bowel into an adjacent part of the bowel. Almost 90% of cases of intussusception are ileocolic, but ileoileal and colocolic types do occur.

A. Intussusception can be seen at any age, but is most common in infants 6 to 12 months old.

B. The classic presentation is intermittent abdominal pain and vomiting with blood and mucus in the stools. The classical "currant-jelly" stools are seen in only half the cases, so intussusception must be considered even if stools are normal.

C. A lead point is commonly found in children over 5, but rarely in children under 2 years old. Several structures can serve as a lead point, including a polyp, lymphoma, hematoma from Henoch-Schönlein purpura (HSP) or hemophilia, hemangioma, and duplication cysts.

E. Reduction of an intussusception by barium or air enema can be achieved in about 75% of cases. If these procedures fail to reduce the intussusception, immediate surgery is required. Delays in diagnosis can lead to severe complications including bowel necrosis, bowel perforation, severe gastrointestinal bleeding, sepsis, and shock.

33. **C.** Metatarsus adductus is a very common deformity of the forefoot in which the metatarsals are deviated medially. Most cases will resolve spontaneously without treatment.

A. This orthopedic condition is due to intrauterine molding and is usually bilateral.

B. Treatment depends on the severity of the deformity. In cases where the forefoot can easily be manipulated into the normal position, passive muscle stretching several times a day may help, but most cases resolve without any treatment. There is no reason for orthopedic referral, radiographs, or special shoes in young babies with flexible metatarsus adductus.

D. If the condition has not resolved by the time the baby needs shoes (~9 months), referral to an orthopedist for casting is appropriate. Referral at 2 to 3 months is not indicated.

E. If, on initial exam, the foot is not flexible and the forefoot cannot be moved into the normal position, referral to an orthopedic surgeon for 6 to 8 weeks of casting is indicated. Surgery is not commonly needed at a young age. Metatarsus adductus in children older than 4 to 6 years of age may require operative correction, but this is an unusual situation.

34. **A.** An audiogram demonstrating significant nerve deafness in this patient would support the diagnosis of familial nephritis with deafness. The urine should demonstrate red cell casts and dysmorphic red cells. Familial nephritis in males generally leads to chronic renal failure, which may be insidious and asymptomatic. Blood chemistries are definitely indicated.

B. There is enough evidence by history to move on with an investigation.

C. A renal biopsy will not be indicated if familial nephritis is demonstrated by other investigation.

D. This patient's mother and his uncle will demonstrate nephritic urine (red blood cells and RBC casts). The mode of transmission of familial nephritis with deafness is most often X-linked dominant and rarely autosomal dominant, and the carrier will have hematuria. The female carrier will frequently have silent microscopic hematuria. Males will develop renal failure and progressive nerve deafness. Hematuria in familial nephritis is due to glomerular bleeding, and therefore the red cells present in the urine are generally abnormal in appearance (dysmorphic), indicative of glomerular bleeding. **E.** An ASO titer will not be indicated with the evidence presented.

35. **D.** The x-ray demonstrates a rather typical TB primary complex with a parenchymal infiltrate and regional lymphadenopathy. There is a right upper lobe infiltrate with right hilar adenopathy. This is suspicious for primary TB infection and the child should be admitted to the hospital for AFB collection. In younger children who do not have a productive cough, the collection of early morning NG aspirates upon awakening on 3 consecutive days should be performed.

A. It would not be appropriate to await purified protein derivative (PPD) results in this case. The tuberculin skin test generally is positive 3 weeks to 3 months after the exposure. This patient's x-ray would suggest the inoculation was at least 1 to 2 months ago and is suspicious for active disease. Therefore, the test should be positive. However, about 10% of immunocompetent children will not develop the delayed hypersensitivity for several months.

B. Sputum collection for AFB is reserved for older children and adolescents who generally have a more productive cough.

C. The treatment of TB is with multidrug therapy. The use of INH alone is reserved for patients with TB exposure who have a positive PPD and negative chest x-ray.

E. Simple observation of this patient is not appropriate management.

36. **D.** Acute infectious diarrhea is a very common entity in pediatrics. Causes include bacteria, viruses, parasites, and preformed toxins. A conservative approach is appropriate when there are no underlying medical problems that exist and there is no evidence for invasive disease (bloody stools and/or white blood cells). If oral rehydration is possible then admission to the hospital can be avoided and stool for culture can be sent as an outpatient. Antibiotics are not indicated unless a specific organism is found or unless there are critical medical issues, such as sepsis or immunocompromise.

A, C. Stool studies should be sent and the diagnosis confirmed before antimicrobial or parasitic therapy is initiated.

B. This child is only mildly dehydrated and deserves a trial of oral dehydration therapy before being admitted to the hospital.

E. A health department investigation would be indicated if a sudden epidemic were to occur at the camp.

37. **A.** An audiogram will give objective information regarding hearing and is essential in every evaluation for speech delay.

B, E. Any radiological imaging, particularly a CT of inner ear structures, is not routine or useful in the evaluation of a hearing deficit unless specific physical findings, such as a cholesteatoma, are seen.

C. An EEG will only give brainwave information and not any information regarding hearing.

D. Speech therapists are experts in this area and are highly useful in language acquisition. However, an objective measure of hearing is necessary before any therapy is initiated.

38. | **D.** The treatment of migraines is aimed at prophylaxis and acute symptomatic treatment. Avoidance of inciting factors and the prophylactic use of propranolol have been shown to help prevent further attacks. |

A. Sumatriptan is not approved for use in children.

B. Narcotics have not been proven beneficial in the management of classic migraines.

C. OTC analgesia, such as ibuprofen, and anti-emetics will help with relief during an acute episode but will not prevent further episodes.

E. Effective preventative treatment, as described above, does exist.

39. | **C.** There is no immunoglobulin deposition in minimal change nephrotic syndrome. |

A. Complement levels are normal in minimal change nephrotic syndrome. Other types of immune-mediated nephrotic syndromes may have low serum complement levels as well as complement deposition in the glomeruli.

B. Minimal change nephrotic syndrome is always accompanied by hyperlipidemia, and all of the lipids are elevated, including cholesterol and triglycerides. This is not specific for this type of nephrosis. Nephrotic syndrome consists of edema, proteinuria exceeding more than 2 g/24 hr, hypoalbuminemia, and hyperlipidemia.

D. About 80% of children with minimal change nephrotic syndrome will respond to glucocorticoid therapy.

E. Other terms for this nephrotic syndrome include minimal change nephrosis, nil disease, and lipoid nephrosis. There is generally a lack of abnormal findings on *light microscopy* . The "minimal change" feature is the fusion or effacement of the podocytes of the epithelial cells along the basement membrane seen by *electron microscopy.*

40. | **A.** The most common bacterial cause of pneumonia in this age group is *Streptococcus pneumoniae.* Although viral infections are believed to cause over 80% of the pneumonias in children, the described case has features to suggest bacterial infection: segmental infiltrate, high fever, and localized crackles. |

B. RSV is the most common infecting organism in the lower respiratory tract for children less than 1 year of age, causing mostly bronchiolitis and pneumonia.

C. Children usually have primary pneumonia with *M. tuberculosis* rather than reactivation TB seen in adults; therefore, this could be TB.

D. Although foreign body aspiration can present as a left lower lobe infiltrate, the child is a little older than the usual age (about 2 to 3 years) and the radiographic appearance is more commonly isolated overinflation of the segment partially blocked by the foreign body. Foreign bodies occur on the right side more often than the left side.

E. Pneumococcal pneumonia does lead to parapneumonic effusion and empyema, but in less than 20% of pneumonias. Based on the information given, there is no way to predict whether this patient will develop an effusion or not.

41. **D.** Referral to a urologist is indicated in this patient with cryptorchidism. Atrophy and delayed testicular development can be seen as early as 1 year in an undescended testis. Exploratory laparotomy with orchiopexy would be indicated once the testis is located.

A. Most studies show that a testis that has not descended by 12 weeks is unlikely to do so.

B. Hormone therapy is infrequently successful, and germ cell loss in the cryptorchid testis can occur as early as 6 months.

C, E. MRI, CT, and ultrasound are not reliable in identifying an intra-abdominal testis, as bowel loops and viscera tend to obscure the testis.

42. **E.** The protective equilibrium response results when the child is pushed laterally by an examiner. The child flexes the trunk toward the force in order to regain the center of gravity while at the same time the arm opposite the force extends to protect against a fall. It does not normally appear until 4 to 6 months of age and then persists voluntarily.

A, B, C, D. The other primitive reflexes listed including startle, hand grasp, crossed adductor, and toe grasp are all present at birth and then disappear over the first 15 months of life.

43. **D.** The most likely diagnosis is nickel dermatitis of the abdominal skin due to contact of the abdominal skin with the metal snap on his jeans; this would account for the central abdominal location of the lesion.

A. The lower mid-abdomen is the wrong location for scabies in a 6-year-old child. Scabies lesions are intensely pruritic and often present in the interdiginous areas of the hands and feet, as well as creases of the neck and axillae.

B. HSP lesions are purpuric, not polymorphous macules, by definition, and are often located on the lower extremities and areas of dependent pressure.

C. The description of this rash does not fit well with poison ivy, especially the central lesion. Poison ivy contact usually occurs on the extremities.

E. Psoriatic lesions are red with a silvery scale and typically present on the extensor surfaces. However, they can sometimes present on the flexor surfaces or central location as described in this scenario.

44.

> **B.** This patient's examination is typical of allergic rhinitis. The allergic gape (continuous open-mouth breathing) and allergic shiners (dark circles under eyes) are classic findings. Patients may also demonstrate an "allergic salute," an upward rubbing of the nose with an open palm or extended fingers. This maneuver may cause an allergic crease across the bridge of the nose. The watery discharge and nonerythematous mucous membranes are also typical. Many patients with allergic rhinitis will have conjunctival erythema and itching.

A. It is true that children whose mothers smoke heavily are at higher risk for developing allergic rhinitis. Other risk factors include family history of atopy, early introduction of foods, heavy exposure to indoor allergens, and higher socioeconomic group.

C. In allergic rhinitis, eosinophils are seen on the nasal smear.

D. Dog and cat allergens are a major problem. Secretions from saliva and sebaceous secretions can remain airborne for long periods. Children can also carry cat allergen on their clothes, thus exposing allergic patients even in cat-free environments. The only effective measure for evading animal allergens in the home is the removal of pets.

E. Oral antihistamines can be used for patients with mild, intermittent symptoms. Patients with more severe symptoms may require treatment with intranasal corticosteroids. If these are not effective, referral to an allergist for skin testing and possible immunotherapy (allergy shots) is indicated.

45.

> **D.** Only in alopecia areata is the skin characteristically smooth, shiny, not scaly, and devoid of broken hairs.

A, B, C, E. Tinea capitus, traction alopecia, trichotillomania , and contact dermatitis to a hair product would all show broken-off hairs and irritation of the skin.

46.

> **D.** The child described in the vignette has congenital hypothyroidism. Its incidence approximates 1 in 4000 and is nearly universally screened for in the United States with newborn screening programs. If children receive treatment by 1 month of age IQ is usually normal, but if treatment is delayed beyond 3 months then IQ can fall below 70. Symptoms of congenital hypothyroidism can include feeding problems, constipation, prolonged jaundice, enlarged posterior fontanelle, tongue thrust, and a hoarse cry.

A, B, C. Abdominal radiograph, CBC, blood culture, and barium swallow studies would all be normal and not aid in the diagnosis of hypothyroidism.

E. Admission to the hospital for an FTT evaluation and monitoring of nutritional status would not yield a diagnosis unless thyroid function tests are obtained.

47.

> **E.** The rash shown in the photo is typical of erythema infectiosum, also called fifth disease. In normal children, this is a mild self-limited illness caused by parvovirus B19. Generally no treatment is needed and no postexposure prophylaxis is required.

A. Amoxicillin is not indicated in the treatment of fifth disease.

B. Immunocompromised children and children with chronic hemolysis may develop anemia, bone marrow suppression, chronic infection, and intense viremia. Such children should not attend school and should avoid exposing pregnant women to the virus. An infected fetus can develop bone marrow suppression, heart failure, hydrops, and/or death.

C. IVIG has been used to treat some immunosuppressed patients with chronic viremia and bone marrow suppression.

D. There is no parvovirus vaccine available.

48. **D.** Polycystic ovarian syndrome (PCOS) is characterized by anovulation and menstrual irregularities and signs of androgen excess such as facial hair, acne, and elevated androgens (DHEA-S, testosterone).

A. Hypothyroidism can cause dysfunctional uterine bleeding and menstrual irregularities with a resultant elevated TSH and low free T4 level.

B. Elevated levels of testosterone would be expected.

C. An elevated LH/FSH ratio would be suggestive of PCOS.

E. Patients with PCOS frequently are hyperlipidemic and more than 50% develop insulin resistance characterized by AN on exam.

49. **E.** The majority of dysfunctional uterine bleeding in adolescents is due to anovulatory cycles from an immature hypothalamic-pituitary-ovarian axis; 50% to 75% of their cycles are anovulatory from menarche to 2 years after menarche.

A. Pregnancy is always a consideration with irregular menstrual bleeding and urine human chorionic gonadotropin (HCG) should be checked. If suspicion is high in a sexually active adolescent and the urine HCG is negative then a quantitative serum HCG should be obtained.

B. ITP typically presents with petechia, bruising, and significant thrombocytopenia following a viral illness. It is more common in younger children.

C. Cervical polyps can occur in adolescents but typically present with intermittent vaginal bleeding.

D. A foreign body, such as a retained tampon, should always be considered with abnormal vaginal bleeding.

50.

> **G.** Iron replacement should be initiated for 3 months to replace stores while menorrhagia is being controlled. Ibuprofen can be used to decrease menstrual blood loss by up to 50%. Oral contraceptives can be started once daily if there is no active bleeding. A monophasic pill with 35 μg of ethinyl estradiol is preferable and the patient can be cycled for 1 to 3 months. If bleeding is stabilized during that time the OCPs can be discontinued. If the patient is actively bleeding at the time of initiating OCPs, a taper can be given to stop the bleeding: "4-3-2" rule of one pill four times a day for 4 days then one pill three times a day for 3 days then one pill twice a day for two days then one pill a day until withdrawal bleeding occurs; using a monophasic pill is preferable with 35 μg of ethinyl estradiol. Anti-emetics are often required with this regimen. The patient can then be cycled for 3 to 6 months on OCPs and then discontinued. Frequently this is enough for the hypothalamic-pituitary-ovarian axis to mature and the menstrual cycles will normalize.

A. Observation alone is not preferable in this patient because she is already anemic.

B. Iron therapy alone will not be sufficient treatment for this patient with menometrorrhagia.

C. Oral contraceptives alone will not be sufficient treatment for this patient with menometrorrhagia.

D. Ibuprofen alone will not be sufficient treatment for this patient with menometrorrhagia.

E. A blood transfusion would only be required if she was overtly symptomatic from her anemia with tachycardia, hypoxia, shortness of breath, etc. This typically would occur only if her hemoglobin was less than 6 g/dL. A work-up for a bleeding disorder should also be undertaken in those situations, while IV estrogen can be used to stop the vaginal bleeding.

F. See explanations for B and C. The explanation for G lists what constitutes the most appropriate management strategy.

H. See explanations for D and E. The explanation for G lists what constitutes the most appropriate management strategy.

Questions

Setting 2: Office

Your office is in a primary care generalist group practice located in a physician office suite adjoining a suburban community hospital. Patients are usually seen by appointment. Most of the patients you see are from your own practice and are appearing for regular scheduled return visits, with some new patients as well. As in most group practices, you will often encounter a patient whose primary care is managed by one of your associates; reference may be made to the patient's medical records. You may do some telephone management, and you may have to respond to questions about articles in magazines and on television that will require interpretation. Complete laboratory and radiology services are available.

51. A 5-month-old infant has been referred to a pediatric cardiologist by you for a murmur suspicious for a ventral septal defect (VSD) found during a well-child checkup. The cardiologist noted that the infant falls on the 25th percentile curves for both height and weight. An echocardiogram done during the office visit confirmed the diagnosis of a small muscular VSD. You discuss the results of the consultation with the mother, who is quite distraught and asks for immediate repair as she had a brother who died from congestive heart failure complications as a child. You calmly explain the defect and the cardiologist's plan of treatment, which seems to set the mother at ease. Which of the following statements would likely be part of that plan?

    A. Cardiac catheterization to confirm the diagnosis and measure the pulmonary artery wedge pressures

    B. Referral to pediatric cardiothoracic surgery for surgical repair at the end of winter viral season

    C. Routine evaluations by the cardiologist with the expectation that the septal defect may close spontaneously

    D. Routine evaluations by the cardiologist with the expectation that the patient will need diuretics and digitalis

    E. NG tube insertion education for the parents, so that increased caloric feeds can be given during the night

---

The next 2 questions (items 52-53) correspond to the following vignette.

A 2-month-old infant presents for his well-child checkup. The mother reports that her child has had a 5-week history of a dry, hacking, persistent cough. He has not had any fevers or other symptoms. The eye discharge she complained about at his 1-month well-child checkup is now gone. His exam shows an afebrile infant with mild retractions and prominent crackles in both lung fields. He has also had poor weight gain, now below the 5th percentile, despite a reliable history of adequate formula intake. Laboratory examination shows a mild elevation in total WBC count with more lymphocytes than neutrophils and a marked eosinophilia. A chest radiograph is obtained (Figure 52).

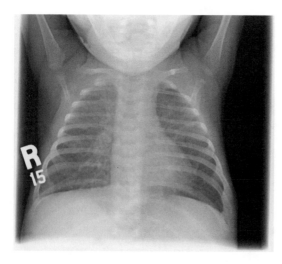

Figure 52 · Image courtesy of the Department of Radiology, Phoenix Children's Hospital, Phoenix, Arizona.

52. Which of the following is the most likely cause of the patient's symptoms?

A. *Streptococcus pneumoniae*
B. Group B streptococcus
C. *Staphylococcus aureus*
D. *Escherichia coli*
E. *Bordetella pertussis*
F. *Chlamydia trachomatis*
G. *Mycoplasma pneumoniae*
H. Herpes simplex
I. Congenital varicella

53. If an infectious work-up were negative, and the mother said the patient's stools were abnormally foul smelling, which of the following metabolic diseases should be considered?

A. Wilson disease
B. Cystic fibrosis (CF)
C. Gaucher disease
D. Galactosemia
E. Hereditary fructose intolerance

End of set

54. You are seeing a 12-month-old HIV-infected child in your office for his 1-year well-child visit. Upon review of his chart you realize that his immunizations are delayed; he has not received any vaccines since 4 months of age. He has a history of multiple ear infections and recurrent pneumonias. His latest labs show an HIV viral load of 25,000 and a CD4 count of 470/14%. Which of the following vaccines should this child receive?

A. Pneumovax
B. *Haemophilus influenzae* vaccine (Hib)
C. Hepatitis A
D. Measles, mumps, rubella (MMR)
E. Varicella

55. A 12-year-old child is being seen in your office for the acute onset of a swollen left testicle. There is no history of trauma. On physical exam you notice an erythematous, swollen, painful left testicle with an absent cremasteric reflex. Which of the following is most consistent with the management of this condition?

A. Surgical consultation should not be delayed
B. Surgical consultation should be deferred pending imaging studies
C. CT scan should be used to confirm the diagnosis
D. Antibiotics are necessary for proper treatment
E. Differentiation from epididymitis is easily demonstrated by exam

56. Two weeks after birth, a girl is brought to your office for evaluation of persistent tearing and a fullness between the eye and the bridge of the nose, just below the medial canthus. The skin over the mass is of normal color, and palpation shows the mass to be soft but yields no discharge. The baby's mother has noted the mass since birth and has noted no changes in its size or appearance. The most appropriate regimen for evaluation and treatment includes:

A. Obtain STAT MRI followed by needle aspiration
B. Request follow-up at 2 years of age, if the tearing persists
C. Hospitalize the child and obtain neurosurgical consultation
D. Request ophthalmology consultation and treatment to occur in the subsequent days
E. Order x-rays of the sinuses and keep the child NPO for a minimum of 24 hours

57. A 13-year-old male is being seen in your office for follow-up of scoliosis. He has been doing relatively well without any complaints. Your partner had been concerned enough to send the patient for radiographs. The report shows the patient has a measured angle of 18° without any other significant pathology noted. The next step in the management of this patient would be:

A. Obtain an MRI for further imaging
B. Referral to an orthopedic surgeon for bracing
C. Referral to an orthopedic surgeon for surgery
D. Continued monitoring every 4 to 6 months
E. No further need to monitor this patient's scoliosis

58. A 4-month-old male infant has been seen on three occasions with febrile illnesses without localizing signs. He is breast fed, and his growth and development have been normal. During weekdays he is in a daycare setting while the mother works, and there are at least five other infants being cared for in that daycare center. The mother is concerned about some sort of immune deficiency that is making her infant susceptible to infections. Which one of the following statements is true?

A. Hypogammaglobulinemia is a normal occurrence at 4 months
B. Infants are born with IgG, IgM, and IgA levels near normal adult values
C. Boys born with X-linked (Bruton) agammaglobulinemia usually develop serious infections before 6 months of age
D. Infants with hypogammaglobulinemia will generally do poorly with ordinary viral infections
E. Patients with hypogammaglobulinemia can usually handle infections with encapsulated organisms normally

59. A 14-year-old girl is seen at your office because of significant pain and swelling of her knees, ankles, and finger joints for the past 6 weeks. She is mildly anemic and has had intermittent fevers, with considerable prostration when she has her fevers. There is no family history of arthritis. There are several subcutaneous nodules found over the extensor surface of her elbows. A rheumatoid factor (RF) is positive, an antistreptolysin O (ASO) titer is negative, her sedimentation rate is 80, and an anti-nuclear antibody (ANA) is significantly positive. Which one of the following statements is true?

A. A positive RF indicates that this girl has IgG antibodies directed against her synovial membranes

B. More than half of patients with this disease will have a positive ANA

C. This type of arthritis occurs equally in males and females

D. Only 10% of these patients will go on to have significant disease as adults

E. The positive ANA strongly suggests that this girl has lupus

60. A 16-year-old female, last seen in your office 9 months ago, now presents with a 15-pound weight gain and complaints of amenorrhea for 3 months. Menarche occurred at 12 years of age and her periods have been regular until 7 months ago. Her flow decreased and she would have a period every 6 to 8 weeks. She also notes that her stools have been hard for the last 6 weeks and improved with Metamucil daily. On further questioning she describes dry skin and a decreased energy level but has a normal affect. What lab test is most likely to render a diagnosis in this patient?

A. CBC

B. Urine β-HCG

C. FSH level

D. Prolactin level

E. TSH

61. You are seeing a 15-month-old boy for a well-child checkup in the office. His mother is concerned about his development. "He is not like the other kids. All of his other friends are cruising and walking already," she states. Which of the following motor milestones should this boy have mastered?

A. Sitting alone

B. Rolling over

C. Cruising

D. Pulling to a stand

E. Walking three steps alone

F. Sitting alone, rolling over, cruising, pulling to a stand, and walking three steps alone

G. Sitting alone and rolling over only

H. Sitting alone, rolling over, and cruising only

I. Sitting alone, rolling over, cruising, and pulling to a stand only

62. You are seeing a 10-year-old female in your office for follow-up of Graves disease. You are discussing the variety of treatment options available for Graves disease with the family. When considering the use of radioactive iodine (^{131}I) therapy for Graves disease in children, it is important to remember the following true statement:

A. Surgical thyroidectomy has a better cure rate than ^{131}I

B. Treatment with methimazole or propylthiouracil (PTU) offers a better long-term remission rate and a low incidence of adverse reactions

C. Surgical thyroidectomy is simple in comparison, and of low risk to the patient

D. ^{131}I has never been used in children

E. ^{131}I is a successful therapy for childhood Graves disease

63. A 15-year-old Jewish girl comes to your office following a recent hospitalization. She was admitted for a history of bruising, nosebleeds, fatigue, and intermittent severe leg pain. On physical exam she has marked hepatosplenomegaly. Laboratory evaluation demonstrates anemia and thrombocytopenia, but the leukocyte count and peripheral smear is normal. A liver biopsy was performed (Figure 63), which shows cells with a "wrinkled paper" appearance. What is the most appropriate next step in the management of this patient?

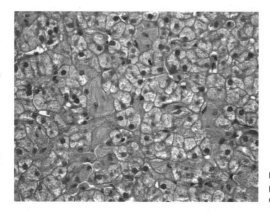

Figure 63 • Image courtesy of the Department of Pathology, Phoenix Children's Hospital, Phoenix, Arizona.

A. Tell the parents that this is an untreatable hereditary condition
B. Measure the acid β-glucosidase activity
C. Initiate therapy with corticosteroids
D. Initiate treatment protocol for acute lymphoblastic leukemia (ALL)
E. Initiate enzyme replacement therapy

64. You are seeing a 10-year-old boy in your office who presents with the sudden onset of unilateral facial weakness and mouth droop. You suspect that he is suffering from a Bell palsy. His mother is concerned about how this will affect his future. Which of the following best describes the prognosis?

A. Most cases result in permanent facial nerve paralysis
B. Twenty-five percent of cases resolve spontaneously with no residual facial weakness
C. Eighty-five percent of cases resolve spontaneously with no residual facial weakness
D. Fifty percent of patients are left with residual facial weakness
E. Fifty percent of cases resolved spontaneously with no residual facial weakness

65. You are seeing a 13-year-old girl who was diagnosed with anorexia nervosa at age 12. She is being managed with antidepressants, counseling with a psychologist, and consultation with a nutritionist. She has a contract with her parents to reward appropriate eating behavior with expanded privileges. Her weight for height has been stable at 19% below ideal body weight for the past 6 months. Today, her weight is at 22% below ideal body weight. She reports no suicidal ideation and her parents agree that she has appeared compliant with the diet and exercise contract. What is the appropriate next step?

A. Contact her psychologist to reevaluate her antidepressant regimen
B. Strengthen the behavior contract to include an increase in caloric intake
C. Admit her to the hospital for nutritional rehabilitation
D. Maintain the current management regimen and reevaluate in 2 weeks
E. Maintain the current management regimen and reevaluate in 1 month

66. You are preparing to perform a circumcision on a 2-week-old infant when you notice an undescended testicle and hypospadias. What is the next step in diagnosis and management?

A. Further genetic and endocrine evaluation
B. Surgical repair of hypospadias
C. Review of newborn screen for inborn errors of metabolism
D. Renal ultrasound
E. Perform circumcision and reevaluate in 2 weeks

67. You are caring for a 6-month-old baby with chronic cough. You order a sweat chloride test and the results show the chloride is 104 mmol/L (normal is < 40) on the right arm and 108 mmol/L on the left arm (with adequate volume of sweat at each site). The next appropriate step is:

A. Repeat the sweat test for confirmation and refer to your local CF center
B. Refer to a geneticist for further evaluation
C. Obtain a stool elastase
D. Send a hair sample for analysis of mineral deficiency
E. Repeat the sweat test in 6 months to confirm the diagnosis

68. You receive a call from a nurse at a local high school about a football player who has been practicing in hot, humid weather and now has become confused and combative. His temperature is measured at 41°C. You are concerned about heat stroke. What advice will you give the nurse for initial management until the patient can be brought to the ED?

A. Give a double dose of aspirin
B. Avoid giving oral and IV fluids
C. Sponge the boy with lukewarm water
D. Remove the boy's clothes and let the body temperature fall slowly
E. Give ice water bath; administer large amount of IV/oral fluids

69. You are seeing a family for a prenatal consult. The mother is 20-weeks pregnant and has been referred secondary to an abnormally low alpha-fetoprotein (AFP) level. Her pregnancy has otherwise been uncomplicated. Which of the following is/are associated with low levels of maternal AFP?

A. Neural tube defects
B. Twin gestation
C. Trisomy 21
D. Gastroschisis
E. Cystic hygroma
F. Neural tube defects and twin gestation
G. Gastroschisis and cystic hygroma
H. Trisomy 21 and cystic hygroma

70. An 8-year-old girl comes to your office because she has been having episodes where she stops moving and talking, demonstrates a blank facial expression, and rapidly blinks her eyelids. These episodes last about 5 to 15 seconds, after which she returns completely to her normal behavior. A true statement about this form of epilepsy is:

A. The episodes can often be induced by hyperventilation for 3 to 4 minutes
B. The typical EEG pattern is called hypsarrhythmia
C. It usually starts in children less than 5 years old
D. These seizures rarely occur more than once a day
E. This type of seizure is commonly treated with dilantin

71. A 10-year-old boy is seen in your office because of complaints of shortness of breath, cough, and fatigue associated with exercise. The patient has a history of reactive airway disease and has been hospitalized twice in the past year for wheezing episodes. You find that on office spirometry, his forced expiratory volume 1 (FEV1) falls by 15% after 7 minutes of heavy exercise. How will you manage this patient initially?

A. Try to minimize strenuous exercise as much as possible
B. Try to exercise mostly when the air is cold
C. Pretreat with albuterol inhaler prior to all exercise
D. Start an inhaled corticosteroid on a twice-daily basis
E. Start oral antihistamines

72. A 9-year-old boy comes to your office because of nightly bedwetting. He has had this problem since he was a very young child and has never had any prolonged period of dryness at night. He has no history of urinary tract infection. Examination of his external genitalia is normal. He reports a normal urinary stream. The boy's father also wet his bed until he was 10 years old. The treatment that most likely will result in a long-term cure is:

A. Strict fluid restriction prior to bed
B. Behavior modification with star charts and rewards
C. Imipramine
D. Desmopressin
E. Buzzer alarm bladder conditioning device

73. A 2-year-old is brought to your office because she has not been moving her arm since yesterday. Last night, she was taken to a local hospital emergency room where an x-ray of her arm proved to be normal. The mother does not remember any trauma, except that the child tripped yesterday while holding hands and walking with her mother. Examination does not reveal joint effusion or point tenderness, but the child will not bend the elbow. What would be the most appropriate next step in management?

A. Repeat the radiographs of the arm
B. Obtain a CT scan of the elbow
C. Prescribe warm soaks and anti-inflammatory agents
D. Refer the patient to an orthopedic surgeon
E. Perform a maneuver to reduce an elbow dislocation

74. A 3-year-old boy was treated in your office with amoxicillin for right otitis media 2 weeks ago. When he returns for an ear check, you find that his tympanic membrane is retracted and there is some clear fluid with air bubbles behind the drum. His mother reports that there has been a mild problem with his hearing. How will you manage this patient?

A. Refer to otolaryngologist
B. Prescribe an oral decongestant medication
C. Prescribe an antibiotic with wider coverage than amoxicillin
D. Have an audiologist perform an audiogram
E. No treatment now, but see patient again in 1 month

75. A mother calls you at 2 AM to report her 3-year-old child has developed a fever of 38.5°C and rash over the past 3 to 4 hours. The rash is described as "little red dots." On further questioning the mother tells you the pinpoint dots appear more red than pink. Some of them are flat and some are raised. Most dots disappear when compressed, but others do not. You suspect that the most likely diagnosis is a nonspecific viral rash. What is the most appropriate advice to give to this child's mother?

A. Antipyretic for fever, no treatment for rash
B. Antipyretic for fever; see patient in office tomorrow
C. Antipyretic for fever, calamine lotion for rash
D. Tell mother to take child to the ED immediately
E. No antipyretic if child is comfortable; see patient in office tomorrow

76. You have been following a 3-year-old patient with atopic dermatitis. You have tried a low-potency steroid cream and some lubrication lotion. The parents return with the concern that the rash is no better and has actually been spreading to new areas. The child has been itching and crying at night. Which of the following would you change to make the family's treatment of the child's atopic dermatitis more effective?

A. Twice daily soaking followed by lubrication
B. Application of emollient followed by a low- to mid-potency steroid cream several times daily
C. Wearing soft, nonirritating clothing
D. Prescription of an antihistamine at bedtime in high enough dosage to cause somnolence
E. Washing only soiled areas of skin with mild, creamed, nonperfumed soap

77. A 12-month-old male infant with tetralogy of Fallot is seen at your office for a presurgical checkup. He has been doing rather well with a minimal number of "blue spells" and surgery is anticipated in a week or two. He is at the 5th percentile for height, and below the 5th percentile for weight. His blood count is as follows: Hb 17.2 g/dL; RBC 5.7; reticulocyte count 1.7%; MCV 66; MCHC 32; MCH 30; and RDW 17.0. Which one of the following is the most important next step in his management?

A. A dietary consultation emphasizing the importance of adequate caloric intake
B. Call the surgeon and recommend immediate surgery
C. Do a partial exchange to reduce the circulating RBCs
D. Immediately begin oral iron therapy
E. Clear this infant for surgery if the extracardiac examination is unremarkable

78. On a routine well-child checkup on a new patient to your practice, you note this 2-year-old girl to have a small hemangioma located over her sacral area in the midline. There is no dimple or hair tufts associated with the lesion. You would recommend for the parents to:

A. Not worry—these lesions usually disappear by age 8
B. Obtain a biopsy of the lesion to rule out a malignant lesion
C. Have the lesion removed by laser treatment to prevent any bleeding or cosmetic problems in the future
D. Get an ultrasound or MRI of the lumbosacral spine to rule out a tethered cord or spinal dysraphism
E. Do nothing, unless the lesion changes in size, color, or thickness

79. A 6-month-old infant boy is seen in your office with failure to thrive. There is a history of child abuse and nutritional deprivation. Your examination reveals significant loss of subcutaneous tissue, growth retardation, and a rachitic rosary is apparent. You make the clinical diagnosis of rickets, and you assume it is secondary to vitamin D deficiency. Regarding this patient, which one of the following will most likely be found?

A. The serum calcium will be normal and phosphorus will be high
B. Alkaline phosphatase will be normal
C. Parathyroid hormone (PTH) will be low
D. Craniotabes may be present in this infant
E. 25 (OH) vitamin D (calcidiol) will be normal

80. A 5-year-old boy is found to have a blood pressure of 120/85. You consult the table of blood pressure norms and find that the 95th percentile for his age and height for systolic and diastolic are 111 and 72, respectively. His physical exam is normal. The blood pressure readings by ambulatory monitoring range between 115 and 125 systolic, and between 80 and 85 diastolic. This blood pressure is consistent with which one of the following?

A. Hypertension
B. High normal blood pressure
C. White coat hypertension
D. Cushing syndrome
E. Adrenogenital syndrome due to 21-hydroxylase deficiency

81. As part of a routine checkup, you order a complete blood count on a 15-month-old African-American boy. His physical exam is normal but he is found to have a hemoglobin level of 8.5 g/dL and a mean corpuscular volume of 66 fL. The lab calls to inform you that red blood cells appear to be abnormal. His blood smear is shown (Figure 81). The next step in this child's management should be:

A. Order a serum ferritin level, obtain a dietary history, and initiate oral ferrous sulfate
B. Perform a lead mobilization test with calcium EDTA
C. Order a hemoglobin electrophoresis for α-thalassemia trait
D. Measure the serum folate level
E. Admit the patient to the hospital for packed red blood cell transfusion

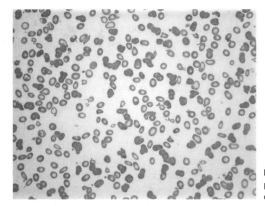

Figure 81 • Image courtesy of the Department of Pathology, Phoenix Children's Hospital, Phoenix, Arizona.

82. A 2-year-old boy with an unrepaired ventricular septal defect (VSD) is going to the dentist to have a dental cavity filled. The dentist asks your advice regarding endocarditis prophylaxis. The best advice would be:

    A. No prophylaxis is necessary
    B. Amoxicillin 50 mg/kg/dose every 6 hours on the day prior to the procedure
    C. Amoxicillin 50 mg/kg/dose, one dose given 1 hour prior to the procedure
    D. Amoxicillin 50 mg/kg, one dose given 3 hours after the procedure
    E. Sulfisoxazole 50 mg/kg/dose, 1 hour before and 1 hour after the procedure

83. A 6-month-old boy is seen in your office because of atopic dermatitis refractory to standard therapy, and only partially responsive to topical steroids. There is a history of prolonged bleeding from his newborn circumcision, and he has had some intermittent bloody diarrhea. He has also had two bouts of otitis media in the past 2 months. Which one of the following disorders is likely to apply to this patient?

    A. Wiskott-Aldrich syndrome
    B. Ataxia telangiectasia
    C. X-linked agammaglobulinemia
    D. Severe combined immunodeficiency
    E. Hyper-IgM syndrome

84. A 9-year-old boy comes to your office for evaluation of "attention problems" at school. Parents report that he has never had difficulty at school before this year, but is now at risk for failing 4th grade due to his disruptive behavior and refusal to complete his schoolwork. He has been in two fights at school and has recently shown a tendency to dangerously impulsive behavior at home. His parents do not recall any previous problems with behavior or any recent illness. Which of the following would probably be most helpful for this child?

    A. Trial of stimulant medication such as methylphenidate (Ritalin)
    B. Testing for learning disabilities
    C. Psychological evaluation for depression or other psychiatric disorder
    D. Thyroid testing
    E. Continued observation and reevaluation in 4 to 6 months

85. You are evaluating a 5-year-old Hispanic girl with Turner syndrome. Her physical exam reveals no evidence of heart murmur, but is significant for a webbed neck, low hairline, and wide-spaced nipples. Which of the following hormonal abnormalities would be expected and necessitate treatment at this time?

A. Low insulin growth factor-1 (IGF-1)
B. Low insulin-like growth factor binding protein 3 (IGFBP3)
C. Estrogen deficiency
D. Growth hormone resistance
E. Adrenocorticotropic hormone (ACTH) deficiency

86. A 1-year-old boy has growth failure over the past several months. Both his weight and height are now below the 5th percentile. Your exam is unremarkable with the exception of his small stature. You decide to investigate the cause of his growth failure. A blood count is unremarkable. Serum electrolytes are Na^+ 140 mEq/L; K^+ 2.5 mEq/L; and Cl^- 117 mEq/L; CO_2 is 12 mEq/L. Serum calcium is 9.0 mg/dL (normal is 8–10 mg/dL) and phosphorus is 2.0 mg/dL. In further investigation, you would expect which one of the following?

A. Significant hypoglycemia
B. Aminoaciduria
C. Elevated BUN and creatinine
D. Urine pH above 6.0
E. Hyperparathyroidism

87. A 15-year-old female presents to your office requesting oral contraceptive pills (OCPs). You counsel her on the complications, benefits, and side effects of OCP usage, which includes which of the following?

A. Increased incidence of anemia
B. Worsening of acne
C. Decreased risk of ovarian cancer
D. Increased risk of endometrial cancer
E. Decreased venous thrombosis

88. A 2-year-old boy who had been walking normally since age 12 months has been noted to have a progressively worsening waddling gait. He falls frequently, has difficulty climbing stairs, and trouble getting up from the floor. On physical exam you note lumbar lordosis and a rubbery feel to his calf muscles. You suspect Duchenne muscular dystrophy. Which of the following is the most accurate information to give to the parents?

A. Enlargement of the calves (pseudohypertrophy) is a classic feature
B. Gross motor skills are often delayed by 2 months of age
C. The creatinine kinase (CK) level becomes elevated at about 2 to 3 years of age
D. The disease affects boys and girls equally
E. The muscle degeneration and fibrosis causes muscle spasms and severe myalgias

89. A 5-year-old boy presents with a history of fever and dysuria. He has a history of having had a urinary tract infection (UTI) when he was 2 years old. He was treated then with an antibiotic and has had no further trouble until now. No investigation was carried out when he had his first UTI. A urinalysis now indicates that he, indeed, has a UTI. There is significant pyuria, and a mid-stream urine grew more than 100,000 *E. coli*. Which one of the following statements is true?

A. It is an acceptable standard to wait for the second UTI in a boy before further urologic investigation
B. UTI often causes significant vesicoureteral reflux
C. Reflux nephropathy rarely leads to end-stage renal disease in children
D. Reflux nephropathy can cause significant hypertension
E. There is no familial incidence of vesicoureteral reflux

90. The parents of a 3-year-old faithfully follow your prescribed treatment for atopic dermatitis. However, the anticubital areas remain wet, weepy, erythematous, and crusted. Which of the following is the most likely explanation for treatment failure in this patient?

A. Secondary bacterial infection
B. Bathing with tepid water
C. Application of steroid cream before the emollient
D. Cool, humid ambient temperatures
E. Excessive use of lubrication

91. You are seeing a 14-year-old boy with prune belly syndrome in your office who has developed chronic renal failure over the past 5 years. Which of the following metabolic abnormalities associated with untreated chronic renal failure is a common finding?

A. Microcytic anemia
B. Delayed bone age
C. Osteosclerosis
D. Hypoparathyroidism
E. Hyperosmolar urine

92. A 17-year-old sexually active female presents to your office with vaginal discharge. The discharge is white and cottage cheese-like and she complains of pruritis. Vaginal pH is less than 4.5 and KOH prep reveals pseudohyphae. Which of the following is the most appropriate therapy?

A. Sitz baths
B. Metronidazole vaginal gel for 5 days
C. Azithromycin 1-g single dose
D. Fluconazole 150-mg single oral dose
E. Metronidazole 2-g single oral dose

93. A 7-year-old female has been evaluated by her pediatrician for short stature and chronic diarrhea. She has not been out of the country and there have been no identified infectious causes. The lab calls her physician with positive anti-transglutaminase and anti-gliadin antibodies suggestive of gluten-sensitive enteropathy (celiac disease). Which of the following is true?

A. There is an increased risk of diabetes type I in this patient
B. There is a higher risk of malignancy with a gluten-free diet
C. Polycythemia is likely to be found on initial labs
D. Often there is a recent exposure to carpet-cleaning solutions
E. The albumin level will be increased

94. A 20-month-old male presents to your office with 5 days of fever to 104°F that reduces minimally with antipyretics. On exam he has a strawberry tongue, edema of the hands and feet, and an erythematous maculopapular rash on his trunk. Which of the following is required to make the diagnosis of Kawasaki disease?

   A. Inguinal lymphadenopathy greater than 2 cm
   B. Nonexudative bulbar conjunctival injection
   C. Oral ulcerations
   D. Mitral valve regurgitation on ECHO
   E. Scrotal edema

The next 2 questions (items 95-96) correspond to the following vignette.

A 15-year-old male calls his coach's wife, a pediatrician, after the development of some chest discomfort, palpitations, near syncope, and dyspnea while in football practice. The symptoms subsided shortly after discontinuation of exercise and he is calling from the locker room. He is feeling ok at this time. The adolescent is in excellent shape and takes no medication. He has a brother with reactive airway disease, but no other problems in the family are reported.

95. Which of the following advice would be most appropriate?

   A. Take two puffs of the brother's albuterol inhaler and call back if no improvement
   B. Lay down on the ground with legs elevated for 15 minutes
   C. Make an appointment with the office next week and avoid exercise until that time
   D. Call his parents so that they can pick him up and take him to be evaluated by a physician today
   E. Take his pulse the next time one of these episodes occurs

96. As the adolescent in the previous case hangs up the phone, a smoke alarm sounds and there is a rush to exit the locker room. While trying to exit, the adolescent slips on some water and falls with hands outstretched on the concrete. There is an obvious fracture of the wrist and the boy is transported via ambulance to the ED where he meets his parents. The ED physician orders a chest x-ray and an ECG along with the casting supplies. On examination the physician notes a heart rate of 100 along with a sharp upstroke of the brachial pulses and a late systolic ejection murmur that increases with standing and decreases with squatting. As you are the patient's primary care physician, the ED physician refers him to your office for follow-up treatment. While reviewing the case history, you note that which of the following statements is most likely to be true?

   A. Albuterol would have had beneficial effects in this case
   B. ECG demonstrates left ventricular hypertrophy
   C. ECG demonstrates supraventricular tachycardia (SVT)
   D. Echocardiogram and CXR shows dextrocardia
   E. Digitalis is frequently used for this problem

End of set

97. An 18-year-old African-American male is seen before leaving for college. He has been healthy throughout his life and takes no medications. Currently he has been having some diarrhea with abdominal cramping and flatulence. He is beginning a weight program for football practice in the fall and as such has been drinking a high-protein milkshake twice daily. He thinks this coincides with the start of his symptoms. When questioned he relates that his mother never drinks milk but she does have some occasional ice cream. Which of the following would be appropriate information to give to this patient?

A. Complete elimination of milk products is needed for symptom relief
B. African-Americans are the most commonly affected individuals
C. Diarrhea is caused by an enzyme deficiency which interferes with NaCl channels
D. Calcium supplements will often cause similar symptoms in these individuals
E. A breath hydrogen study can confirm the diagnosis, but often an appropriate dietary change is all that is needed

98. A newborn male infant is seen shortly after birth. The diagnosis of trisomy 21 is considered and a genetics consult is ordered. The geneticist evaluates the infant the next day and concurs with the diagnosis. High-resolution chromosomes are sent. Nursing reports that there have not been any problems except that there has been no passage of meconium. The anus appears patent. Of the following, which is the most likely reason for the lack of stooling?

A. Congenital hypothyroidism
B. Duodenal atresia
C. Hirschsprung disease
D. Meckel diverticulum
E. Tracheoesophageal fistula (TEF)

The next 2 questions (items 99-100) correspond to the following vignette.

The best-corrected visual acuity of the right eye of a 7-year-old boy is noted to be 20/20, while that of his left eye is 20/200. His pupils are equal in size and reactivity. The left eye drifts inward.

99. The most appropriate therapeutic regimen should include:

A. Wait until puberty to begin therapy
B. Begin patching the right eye immediately
C. Advise the parents that their son is too old to begin therapy
D. Patch the left eye each night at bedtime
E. Urgent surgery to realign the eyes

100. After detailed description of the disease process, you should ensure a follow-up appointment to reassess the visual acuity within:

A. One day
B. Two weeks
C. Three months
D. Four years
E. Follow-up evaluation is not indicated

End of set

Answers and Explanations

Answer Key

51. C	68. E	85. D
52. F	69. C	86. B
53. B	70. A	87. C
54. B	71. D	88. A
55. A	72. E	89. D
56. D	73. E	90. A
57. D	74. E	91. B
58. A	75. D	92. D
59. B	76. B	93. A
60. E	77. D	94. B
61. I	78. D	95. D
62. E	79. D	96. B
63. B	80. A	97. E
64. C	81. A	98. C
65. C	82. C	99. B
66. A	83. A	100. C
67. A	84. C	

51. **C.** In an otherwise healthy infant with a small VSD, no invasive therapy or surgical intervention is needed immediately. However, close monitoring and subacute bacterial endocarditis (SBE) prophylaxis is indicated. Spontaneous closure is likely with small VSDs and muscular VSDs. Often there is a history of congenital defects in the family.

A. Cardiac catheterization would not be indicated in this scenario, but is useful in helping to manage those patients with complex congenital lesions.

B. As in the explanation for C, spontaneous closure is likely with a small muscular VSD; surgery is not necessary in this scenario.

D. The patient should periodically be followed for spontaneous closure, but the likelihood of developing congestive heart failure from a small VSD is rare.

E. This patient is growing well at the 25th percentile and does not need NG feeds. NG feeds for caloric supplementation would be indicated in cases of poor growth and suboptimal weight gain.

52. **F.** *Chlamydia trachomatis* is the most likely cause of this patient's symptoms, which are quite typical, including dry, hacky, classically described as staccato, cough that started in the first month of life, slow progression over weeks with progressive respiratory distress, afebrile, peripheral eosinophilia, eye discharge, and failure to thrive despite adequate formula intake.

A, B, C, D. The fact that he has had symptoms for several weeks without any fevers makes the more virulent bacterial strains unlikely (Strep, Staph, *E. coli*).

E. Pertussis could cause a cough for a prolonged period and should be considered, but the coughing typically occurs in spasms and is not associated with a peripheral eosinophilia, but a marked lymphocytosis instead.

G. Mycoplasma is a common cause of atypical pneumonia in childhood, but not in infants.

H, I. Herpes simplex and varicella can cause neonatal infections, but they have other associated symptoms, which often will include vesicular skin lesions.

53. **B.** CF is the only metabolic disease listed that could explain the above patient's symptoms, and should be considered in any infant who has respiratory symptoms and failure to thrive, even if there were not a history of foul smelling stools suggestive of fat malabsorption. The various genetic defects in chloride channels that cause CF result in problems with secretions; the systems most affected are the respiratory and gastrointestinal systems. All the other metabolic diseases above are not associated with respiratory problems.

A. Wilson disease affects copper metabolism and presents with liver, neurologic, or psychiatric manifestations much later in childhood.

C. Gaucher disease is a lysosomal storage disease that presents with pathologic fractures, bone pain, hepatosplenomegaly, and/or hematologic problems.

D. Galactosemia comes from an inability to break down galactose found in human and cow's milk and can present in the newborn period with poor weight gain, jaundice, vomiting, irritability, feeding difficulties, or full blown sepsis, often from *E. coli*. However, respiratory distress is not one of its features.

E. Hereditary fructose intolerance presents in infants when they are first fed fruit, fruit juices, or table sugar (sucrose) and symptoms can mimic those of galactosemia. Again, slowly progressive respiratory distress is not part of the clinical picture.

54. **B.** All HIV-infected children without evidence of severe immunosuppression or symptomatology should receive all of the following vaccines by 12 months of age: prevnar, Hib, hepatitis B, DTaP (diphtheria, tetanus, acellular pertussis vaccine), and IPV (inactivated polio vaccine). These are all inactivated vaccines and are recommended to be given to all HIV-infected children regardless of their immune status and CD4 counts.

A. Pneumovax is a 23-valent pneumococcal vaccine that is recommended in children older than 2 years of age who are HIV infected, as well as other selectively immunocompromised or asplenic patients, such as those with sickle cell anemia.

C. Hepatitis A vaccine (HAV) is recommended in high-risk children older than 2 years of age, such as those with HIV, as well as those living in areas with a high prevalence of disease. HAV is also often required before children can be enrolled in Head Start programs.

D, E. As the MMR and varicella vaccines are live attenuated vaccines, they should NOT be given to HIV-infected children who are considered to be severely immunocompromised with CD4 counts less than 15%, such as the child in this scenario.

55. **A.** The clinical scenario of scrotal swelling and pain with absence of the cremasteric reflex is consistent with testicular torsion. Testicular torsion occurs more commonly in children younger than 6 years of age, although it is seen through adolescence as well. Testicular survival decreases rapidly after 6 hours and demonstrates the need for prompt surgical intervention.

B. Ultrasound with Doppler or isotopic scans can be useful in the diagnosis, but should not delay further surgical consultation or intervention.

C. CT scan is expensive and not recommended in this clinical situation.

D. Antibiotics are not indicated in the treatment of testicular torsion.

E. Epididymitis occurs more commonly in adolescence, but can mimic testicular torsion. A urinalysis will often reveal pyuria in the case of epididymitis and the cremasteric reflex should be present.

56. **D.** The diagnosis is dacryocystocele. Tearing and a small mass in the inner corner of the lower eyelid characterize this form of congenital nasolacrimal duct obstruction. It is due to an amniotic fluid distended nasolacrimal sac. In addition to the simpler distal obstruction of most congenital nasolacrimal duct obstructions, a dacryocystocele has a proximal obstruction of the punctae or common canaliculus. Surgical dilatation of the proximal tear system is needed in the first few weeks of life to prevent a life-threatening cellulitis. Distal dilatation can be attempted, but is not always successful.

A. Imaging is not needed in this case. The typical findings of this case are consistent with the diagnosis of a dacryocystocele—congenital, tearing, nonprogressive fullness below the medial canthal tendon. The treatment of choice is opening the proximal tear system, not penetrating the skin.

B. Early diagnosis and treatment is critical for dacryocystocele. Surgical treatment of congenital nasolacrimal duct obstructions is best performed by 1 year, with a 90% cure rate. Surgical treatment of dacryocystocele should be performed in the first year of life.

C. Hospitalization and systemic antibiotic therapy is needed for an infected dacryocystocele, which has the characteristics of this case plus erythema of the skin overlying the nasolacrimal sac, and a purulent discharge. Neurosurgical evaluation would be helpful if the mass was above the medial canthal tendon and shown to connect with the CNS, such as occurs with an encephalocystocele.

E. Imaging is rarely indicated, unless nonclassic signs are present. Just prior to the anesthetic and surgical period, an NPO status can be instituted for 4 to 6 hours.

57. **D.** Curves that measure less than 25° usually do not require any immediate intervention, but should be monitored every 4 to 6 months for continued progression of curvature. Curves that are greater than 25° should be referred to an orthopedic surgeon for further management.

A. Obtaining an MRI in this scenario is unnecessary and expensive. An MRI may be indicated if further pathology were noted on x-ray, such as a compressed disc, or if neurologic symptoms develop.

B. Bracing for scoliosis is typically reserved for patients with curves from 25° to 45°.

C. Surgical intervention is required for correction of curves greater than 45°.

E. The risk of progression of the patient's scoliosis still exists and it would be malpractice to ignore further progression of disease. Of note, premenarchal girls with a curve of 20° or more have a higher risk of disease progression than those with the same curve who are 1 to 2 years postmenarche.

58. **A.** Hypogammaglobulinemia is expected at 3 to 4 months when the maternally derived IgG antibodies reach a nadir, and the infant's own IgG production is not yet optimal. A level as low as 200 mg/dL is not unusual. The occasional infant with a benign "transient hypogammaglobulinemia of infancy" may get as low as 100 mg/dL, but recovery in these infants is seen by 6 to 12 months. Normal adult level of IgG is near 1000 mg/dL.

B. IgG is the smallest immunoglobulin molecule and is readily transferred to the infant in utero. Therefore, infants are born with IgG levels similar to the mother. IgM and IgA, however, do not cross the placenta, and therefore levels of these immunoglobulins are very low in the newborn. Any significant amount of IgM (above 20 mg/dL) in the newborn should make one suspicious of congenital infection.

C. Bruton agammaglobulinemia infants (agammaglobulinemia) generally do well for 6 to 9 months while maternal immunoglobulins are still present. The development of infections with encapsulated organisms becomes problematic in the last half of the first year.

D. Ordinary viral infections generally do not pose problems in infants with agammaglobulinemia, because viral infections are handled more by cellular immune functions. The exceptions are hepatitis viruses and enteroviruses.

E. Those patients with immunoglobulin deficiencies are at increased risk of infection from encapsulated organisms such as *Streptococcus pneumoniae* and *Haemophilus influenzae*.

---

59. **B.** About 75% of older children and adolescents with *RF-positive* rheumatoid arthritis have a positive ANA.

A. RF is an IgM antibody directed against the Fc portion of the patient's own IgG.

C. This patient would be classified as having late-onset polyarticular juvenile rheumatoid arthritis (JRA) with onset of disease after 8 years of age and more than four joints affected. Eighty percent of late-onset polyarticular JRA occurs in girls.

D. Late-onset polyarticular RF-positive JRA acts much like the adult disease. About 50% will go on to have significant and frequently disabling disease.

E. The likelihood of lupus in this patient is remote if there is no other confirmatory evidence clinically or by further testing. In late-onset RF-positive JRA, ANA is positive in about 75% of patients.

---

60. **E.** This patient's constellation of symptoms is classic for hypothyroidism. She has decreased energy, constipation, weight gain, and amenorrhea. TSH will be elevated with a decreased T4 level.

A. A CBC would be useful in evaluating for anemia with symptoms of fatigue, but there is no history of heavy menstrual bleeding or other symptoms to suggest the patient may be anemic.

B. A urine β-HCG should be obtained on all patients with secondary amenorrhea, but pregnancy does not explain the remainder of her symptoms.

C. FSH levels are helpful for evaluating primary ovarian failure and will be elevated.

D. A prolactin level is elevated in patients with pituitary microadenomas who may present with amenorrhea but frequently have galactorrhea. They may also demonstrate visual field defects on neurologic exam, and an MRI of the brain should be obtained.

---

61. **I.** The boy in this scenario should have mastered the following skills by 15 months of age: sitting alone, rolling over, cruising, and pulling to a stand. His mother should not be concerned at this point if he has mastered these skills. Table 61 represents the ranges of normal development for the above-listed tasks. Notice that this 15-month-old child is still within the normal range of development even if he is still not walking independently.

A, B, C, D, E, F, G, H. See explanation for I.

■ TABLE 61	Normal Motor Milestones Development Ranges
Rolling over	2 to 5 months
Sitting alone	5 to 7 months
Pulling to a stand	7 to 9 months
Cruising	8 to 13 months
Walking three steps alone	9 to 17 months

62.   **E.** ^{131}I is a controversial but successful therapy for childhood Graves disease. Radioactive ^{131}I has been used to treat children with Graves disease; in fact, it has been used in children as young as 1 year of age. It is a simple, inexpensive, and efficacious therapy (> 90% cure rate) that is rarely accompanied by acute side effects. However, long-term studies do not exist, so long-term risks have not been adequately assessed.

A, C. Surgical thyroidectomy offers a similar cure rate to ^{131}I (around 90% if performed by a skilled thyroid surgeon), but has greater immediate risk and cost.

B. PTU and methimazole are commonly used therapies for children with Graves disease; however, both drugs offer a *low* long-term remission rate (< 30% to 40%) and a *high* incidence of adverse reactions (20% to 30%), which may be (rarely) fatal.

D. As in the explanation for E, ^{131}I has been used successfully in children.

63.   **B.** The liver biopsy demonstrates the classic Gaucher cell, engorged with glucocerebroside, giving a "wrinkled paper" appearance. Gaucher disease is the most common lysosomal storage disease and is often seen in Ashkenazi Jews. The condition is due to a deficient activity of acid β-glucosidase, with resultant deposition of glycolipids in cells of the reticoendothelial system. The progressive deposition causes infiltration of the bone marrow, progressive hepatosplenomegaly, and skeletal complications. The liver biopsy findings strongly suggest Gaucher disease, but similar cells can be seen in granulocytic leukemia and myeloma; therefore, suspected cases should be confirmed by measuring acid β-glucosidase activity in leukocytes or cultured fibroblasts.

C. Corticosteroids have no roll in the treatment of Gaucher disease.

D. A bone marrow analysis would be expected to show greater than 30% leukemic lymphoblasts to make the diagnosis of ALL; these lymphoblasts would also be expected to be seen on peripheral smear. This patient, however, has Gaucher disease.

A, E. Gaucher disease can be treated with enzyme replacement therapy with IV infusion of recombinant acid β-glucosidase. The organomegaly and abnormal hematologic abnormalities are reversed initially and then, with monthly maintenance doses, bone pain is decreased and growth improves.

64.   **C.** Bell palsy is an acute facial paralysis caused by facial nerve dysfunction. The etiology is suspected to be viral in a majority of cases. Eighty-five percent of cases will resolve spontaneously with no residual facial weakness.

A, D. Only 5% are left with permanent facial weakness, while another 10% will have minor residual facial weakness.

B, E. As in the explanation for C, 85% of cases resolve spontaneously with no residual facial weakness.

65. | **C.** Admit to the hospital for nutritional rehabilitation and psychiatric care. This child is failing maximal outpatient management of anorexia nervosa. Anorexia nervosa is a life-threatening illness with a mortality rate from 2% to 8%; death usually results from a combination of decreased myocardial muscle mass and electrolyte imbalance. Hospitalization is often indicated once the patient's weight drops to 80% (or below) of their ideal body weight.

A. Antidepressants have not been shown to be markedly helpful in managing anorexia. It is unlikely that a shift in medication will reverse the persistent weight loss and may delay decision making around hospitalization.

B. While both parents and child report compliance with the behavior contract, the persistent weight loss implies that this child is managing to circumvent the contract surreptitiously, a hallmark of anorexic behavior. Changing the contract is unlikely to bring about the desired effect.

D, E. Watchful waiting may bring this child closer to death. She has been in a starvation state for several months already and has failed outpatient management.

66. | **A.** Further genetic and endocrine evaluation for intersexuality/hermaphroditism is indicated. Because hypospadias is an anatomical anomaly of anterior urethral development, boys with simple hypospadias should have otherwise normal genitalia. Patients with ambiguous genitalia, by contrast, have a more extensive genital anomaly, reflecting the failure of all androgen-dependent development. A useful rule of thumb is to assume that any baby with "hypospadias," as well as an undescended testis and/or bifid scrotum, should be investigated for hermaphroditism, with immediate hormonal, chromosomal, and anatomic studies.

B. Surgical repair of the hypospadias will be necessary, but can wait until the genetic evaluation is complete and a decision is made as to whether orchiopexy will be necessary.

C, D. This combination of hypospadias and undescended testicle is not associated with any particular inborn error of metabolism or renal abnormality.

E. Circumcision at this point is not recommended and should be avoided in patients with hypospadias as the foreskin may be needed for future repair.

67. | **A.** A sweat chloride value above 60 mmol/L is diagnostic of CF. Because the test requires precise technical performance, all positives are repeated for confirmation. Subsequent DNA analysis is often obtained as well. CF centers specialize in the care of children with CF and outcomes are generally better when the CF center participates in the child's care.

B. Genetic counseling is appropriate to consider if there is trouble establishing the diagnosis by sweat testing or if there are family-planning issues.

C. Stool elastase may help identify pancreatic insufficiency, but is not diagnostic of CF.

D. Mineral deficiency is not a cause of a positive sweat test nor the cause of CF.

E. Six months is too long to wait to confirm the diagnosis; appropriate therapy will not be initiated if the diagnosis is delayed.

68. **E.** Treatment for heat stroke starts with CPR with attention to the ABCs (airway, breathing, and circulation). These patients may be dehydrated and hypotensive. Aggressive cooling with ice water baths, cooling fans, and removal of excess clothing is required to return the body temperature to normal as quickly as possible. Rapid administration of IV fluids is important for the treatment of hypovolemia; in settings where an IV would be difficult or impossible to place, aggressive oral rehydration should be initiated.

A. Aspirin and other antipyretics work by bringing the body's "thermostat" back to a normal setting. Because the thermostat is not elevated in heat-related illness, aspirin would have no effect on the body temperature in this case.

B. This patient needs rapid administration of fluids.

C, D. Neither lukewarm sponge baths nor removal of clothing will bring the body temperature down fast enough.

69. **C.** Down syndrome, trisomy 21, is associated with low maternal levels of AFP, as are trisomy 18, intrauterine growth retardation, and incorrect gestational age.

A, B, D, E. *High* levels of AFP are associated with conditions such as neural tube defects, twin gestation, gastroschisis, cystic hygromas, and polycystic renal disease. AFP levels are typically drawn during 16 to 18 weeks of gestation to serve as a screening tool for the above-listed conditions.

70. **A.** The episodes described are typical absence (petit mal) seizures. There is no aura and no postictal state. Sometimes teachers mistake the stare and expressionless face for inattentive misbehavior. Hyperventilation can be used in the office setting to induce onset of an episode.

B. The classic EEG pattern of absence seizures shows 3 cycles per second spike-wave complexes. Hypsarrhythmia is seen in infantile spasms.

C. Absence seizures are rare under age 5 and are more common in girls than in boys.

D. Children with absence seizures may have countless seizures during a single day.

E. Absence seizures are commonly treated with ethosuximide (Zarontin), not dilantin.

71. **D.** This patient has exercise-induced asthma (EIA), which is commonly associated with wheezing, cough, shortness of breath, fatigue, and lack of interest in physical activities. The diagnosis is confirmed with a 10% to 15% fall in FEV1 with an exercise challenge. Although EIA is occasionally an isolated illness, the vast majority of patients with this problem also have poorly controlled underlying persistent reactive airway disease. Because this patient has been hospitalized twice in the last year, it is unlikely he has isolated EIA. For both his persistent asthma and the EIA, an inhaled corticosteroid should be prescribed to control airway inflammation.

A. The goal should be normal physical activity. Inactivity or reduced exertion should not be accepted.

B. Cold air tends to make EIA worse.

C. Using inhaled albuterol prior to exercise may be useful for patients with pure EIA who do not have underlying persistent asthma. There is some evidence that the effect of albuterol wears off quickly in many patients.

E. Antihistamines are not indicated in EIA.

72. **E.** Buzzer alarm conditioning devices take several months to decrease the frequency of bedwetting, but they have the best long-term cure rates for primary nocturnal enuresis. These alarms will help approximately 75% to 80% of enuretics to achieve nighttime dryness. In comparison, the spontaneous cure rate even without any treatment is approximately 15% per year.

A. Fluid restriction prior to bed is ineffective.

B. Behavior modification with star charts and rewards for dry nights seems to improve cure rates when used in conjunction with other enuresis treatments.

C, D. Medications, such as imipramine and desmopressin, may help some children; however, once the medicine is discontinued the majority of children relapse. Desmopressin is very expensive. While less expensive, imipramine is a dangerous medication that can cause cardiac arrhythmias and convulsions if overdosed. Many pediatricians reserve medications for special situations such as a slumber party or summer camp.

73. **E.** A nursemaid's elbow (radial head subluxation) is caused by a sudden, forceful pull on an extended forearm. Commonly, this condition occurs when a child trips while holding a parent's hand or when the child is being swung by his or her arms. Immediately following the event, the child refuses to use the arm. The elbow appears normal on physical exam and the x-ray is often normal. The primary care physician can attempt reduction by gently flexing the elbow with the palm up until a palpable snap is felt at the lateral elbow.

A. Radiographs may be needed if there is joint fluid and/or point tenderness that suggest presence of a fracture.

B. A CT scan is expensive and not indicated in this case.

C. Warm soaks and anti-inflammatory agents would delay proper treatment. The longer the elbow stays subluxed, the harder it is to reduce back into the normal position in the joint.

D. Orthopedic consultation would be indicated if the reduction maneuver was not successful. Once the subluxation is reduced, the child will begin using the arm normally almost immediately.

74. E. A retracted tympanic membrane with an effusion in the middle ear and mild hearing loss suggests that the eustachian tube is blocked. This condition is called otitis media with effusion (OME) and is commonly seen for several weeks following a bout of acute otitis media (AOM). In fact, it is so common as to be considered part of the natural course of AOM. This condition is not due to treatment failure and there is no need for additional expensive antibiotics at this time. Furthermore, most studies have failed to show that oral decongestants are efficacious for preventing or treating OME.

A. Referral to an otolaryngologist for placement of tympanostomy tubes should be delayed until the effusion has been present for 4 to 6 months.

B, C. As in the explanation for E, neither amoxicillin nor a decongestant is appropriate or useful for the treatment of OME.

D. Current recommendations suggest that audiology evaluation be considered if OME persists for longer than 6 weeks to 3 months.

75. D. The mother should be instructed to take her child to the emergency room. While a nonspecific viral rash is most likely, you cannot rule out the possibility of meningococcemia. Meningococcal infections in the blood or spinal fluid can be life threatening and require immediate medical attention. Rashes are extremely difficult to diagnose over the phone because parents may have difficulty giving an accurate description of the lesions. Typically, meningococcemia is associated with petechiae, pinpoint spots caused by leakage of blood from capillaries. These lesions are red-purple in color and are either not raised or only slightly raised. When the lesion is compressed or the surrounding skin is stretched, the petechial lesions remain visible. In contrast, a nonspecific viral rash is maculopapular, pink in color, and blanches (disappears) when compressed.

A, B, C. Although antipyretics may be given for fever, the concern for meningococcemia necessitates that the child be evaluated immediately, rather than in the office tomorrow. Calamine lotion would not be indicated.

E. Delay in treatment of this child until tomorrow would be inappropriate in this scenario.

76. B. The steroid cream needs to be applied before the emollient to be effective.

A. Soaking in plain water (not bathing with soap) to hydrate the skin is helpful before application of steroid cream and emollient.

C. Clothing that is nonirritating, such as cotton and certain synthetics, will cause less pruritus.

D. Antihistamine dosages need to be high enough to cause somnolence to be effective in decreasing pruritis.

E. Judicious use of nondrying soaps in limited areas is now accepted.

---

77. | **D.** This is iron deficiency in this infant with cyanotic heart disease. Hypoxemia overdrives the erythropoiesis causing the polycythemia. The microcytosis (low MCV) and high RDW indicate that there is iron deficiency. Iron-deficient RBCs are extremely nondeformable (rigid), increasing blood viscosity. These patients are prone to clot and have strokes. Iron therapy is indicated.

A. Dietary advice would also be indicated because this infant is iron deficient, but it would be more important first to begin iron therapy.

B. There is no surgical urgency as long as this infant is doing well. It is probably wise to correct the iron deficiency before surgery.

C. A partial exchange would only reduce this infant's oxygen-carrying capacity.

E. It would be wise to wait a bit for surgery until the iron therapy at least partially corrects the iron deficiency, as long as there is no urgent need for surgery (at least 3 to 4 weeks). Any episode of dehydration could precipitate a stroke.

---

78. | **D.** Vascular lesions in the midline over the spine can often be associated with spinal and spinal cord abnormalities. These require further imaging to uncover hidden spinal lesions of serious future significance.

A. It is true that many infantile hemangiomas appearing in the first 6 months of life will resolve by 8 years of age. However, further investigation is prudent for ones located over midline structures.

B. A malignant hemangioma is very unlikely. Biopsy also carries some risks of significant bleeding.

C. Investigation for underlying serious pathology should be done before removal of the lesion.

E. Watching for changes is an appropriate approach for nevi and vascular lesions not located in the midline.

---

79. | **D.** Craniotabes is a thinning of the skull seen in rickets causing a "ping pong" effect to palpation. This may be a physical sign of rickets.

A. While serum calcium and phosphorus may be normal early in vitamin D deficiency, both will be low in manifest cases of vitamin D deficiency rickets.

B. Alkaline phosphatase is high in all forms of rickets, indicating increased osteoblast activity.

C. PTH is stimulated by low serum calcium; therefore, in all forms of rickets associated with low calcium, PTH will be high. Thus, this patient with vitamin D deficiency will have an elevated PTH.

E. 20-Hydroxylation of vitamin D takes place in the liver, but in vitamin D deficiency there is lack of substrate, and therefore there will be deficient production of this intermediary product. The most active form of vitamin D (1,25 [OH]$_2$

vitamin D) is produced in the kidney, and this may be normal early, but would be expected to be low in severe cases.

80. **A.** Clearly, the blood pressure readings are consistently over the 95th percentile. This is true hypertension, not just high normal.

B. The blood pressure readings are consistently over the 95th percentile, which defines true hypertension, not just high normal blood pressure. This is confirmed by ambulatory monitoring.

C. White coat hypertension is generally a finding in older children and adolescents, and is ruled out by ambulatory monitoring.

D. While Cushing syndrome is a cause of hypertension, this is not likely in view of the normal physical exam.

E. The adrenogenital syndrome due to 21-hydroxylase deficiency causes salt wasting and does not cause hypertension. It is the adrenogenital syndrome secondary to 11-hydroxylase that has significant sodium-retaining effects and can cause hypertension.

81. **A.** The smear demonstrates microcytic, hypochromic red blood cells, which are typical of iron deficiency anemia. In children, this is most commonly due to inadequate iron intake, often as a result of being fed large amounts of whole milk, which contains little absorbable iron. Patients with iron deficiency anemia have a low MCV and an elevated RDW. The MCV should be at least 70 plus the child's age (in years). Further laboratory evaluation would likely yield an elevated or normal TIBC, and decreased ferritin, iron, and percent saturation.

B. With lead poisoning, basophilic stippling may be seen in peripheral blood cells. Iron deficiency is often seen in association with lead poisoning, so lead screening is important in children living in older housing. A blood lead level would be done prior to consideration of a lead mobilization test (which is done to determine which children are likely to benefit from chelation therapy).

C. In α-thalassemia trait, the MCV is low but the total number of RBCs is elevated with a normal RDW. Hypochromia is not seen on the blood smear, and laboratory evaluation should reveal a normal iron, TIBC, percent saturation, and ferritin. While hemoglobin electrophoresis can detect β-thalassemias, it does not generally detect α-thalassemia trait except in young infants.

D. In folate deficiency, the red cells are larger than normal, resulting in a hyperchromic anemia with an elevated MCV. Folate deficiency is often seen in babies who are fed goat's milk.

E. Dietary iron deficiency anemia can generally be treated as an outpatient. Blood transfusions and hospital admission are usually reserved for patients who have evidence of hemodynamic instability or excessive fatigue secondary to their anemia.

82. **C.** The American Academy of Pediatrics (AAP) recommends that children with congenital heart disease who are undergoing a dental procedure be given antibiotics to prevent endocarditis. The standard prophylaxis regimen is amoxicillin 50 mg/kg, given as a one-time dose an hour before the procedure. Prophylaxis is also recommended for certain respiratory tract, gastrointestinal tract, and genitourinary tract procedures that are likely to cause transient bacteremia. For patients who are allergic to penicillin, the drug of choice is clindamycin.

A. Patients who do *not* require prophylaxis include those with 1) physiologic or innocent murmurs, 2) an isolated secundum atrial septal defect (ASD), 3) a surgically repaired ASD, ventricular septal defect (VSD), or patent ductus arteriosus (PDA), and 4) mitral valve prolapse without valvular regurgitation. This patient, however, does require prophylaxis.

B, D. These are correct dosages, but administered at incorrect times.

E. This is not the standard prophylaxis regimen recommended by the AAP.

83. **A.** This patient probably has Wiskott-Aldrich syndrome, which is an X-linked recessive syndrome consisting of atopic dermatitis, thrombocytopenia, and susceptibility to infection. Patients with Wiskott-Aldrich syndrome have impairment in the formation of antibodies to the polysaccharide capsular antigens. In general IgM is low, IgA and IgE are elevated, and IgG is slightly low.

B. Ataxia telangiectasia is an autosomal recessive syndrome consisting of thrombocytopenia, progressive ataxia, and variable humoral and cellular immunodeficiency.

C. Patients with Wiskott-Aldrich syndrome have impairment in the formation of antibodies to the polysaccharide capsular antigens, but they are not agammaglobulinemic. In general IgM is low, IgA and IgE are elevated, and IgG is slightly low.

D. Severe combined immunodeficiency patients have severe deficiency of both cellular and humoral immunity. Gammaglobulin levels are extremely low to absent, and absolute leukocyte counts are frequently less than 500/μL.

E. Hyper-IgM syndrome is an X-linked immunodeficiency syndrome consisting of elevated polyclonal IgM, and usually normal T-cell function. These patients develop frequent respiratory infections beginning in the first or second year. Lymphoid hyperplasia is usually present.

84. **C.** Psychological evaluation for depression or other psychiatric disorder should be initiated. This child is showing an acute change in behavior, more consistent with anxiety or depression, and should be evaluated before symptoms worsen.

A. While this child is showing some of the hallmark characteristics of attention deficit/hyperactivity, part of the diagnostic criteria for ADHD includes presence of symptoms before age 7.

B. Testing for learning disabilities is also warranted, but the acute nature of his behavior change both at home and at school warrants a careful assessment of mood disorder as the initial evaluation.

D. Hyperthyroidism can mimic psychiatric disorders and should be ruled out, but testing should neither delay nor replace psychological evaluation.

E. Simple observation and reevaluation in the future is not acceptable given the evolving severity of behaviors in this child.

---

85. **D.** Turner syndrome is a chromosomal disorder (gonadal dysgensis: XO) resulting in a syndrome characterized by short stature, lymphedema, webbed neck, low posterior hairline, and cubitus valgus; there are often associated cardiac and renal anomalies as well. Growth hormone (GH) therapy is standard care for a child with Turner syndrome. Its use is not for the treatment of GH deficiency but for the treatment of GH resistance. As a consequence, the dosage of GH used in Turner patients is higher than the patient with GH deficiency. Other associated endocrine conditions in Turner syndrome include glucose intolerance and hypothyroidism. In addition, certain autoimmune disorders are noted in Turner patients, including Hashimoto thyroiditis, celiac disease, inflammatory bowel disease, and JRA.

A, B. Although GH is used in Turner patients, they do not have GH, IGF-1, and IGFBP3 deficiency, and require GH therapy because of GH resistance.

C. Most Turner syndrome patients will have delayed puberty and estrogen deficiency. Estrogen does not cause the short stature seen in these patients. A 5-year-old girl would be prepubertal and not need estrogen replacement therapy until she is older than 12 years of age.

E. ACTH deficiency is not associated with Turner syndrome.

---

86. **B.** The findings of hyperchloremic acidosis and hypophosphatemia with growth delay suggest this patient has Fanconi syndrome. Aminoaciduria is a feature of Fanconi syndrome, which this patient probably has. The aminoaciduria is not selective because there is a generalized proximal tubular dysfunction.

A. Glycosuria is a feature of Fanconi syndrome, which is secondary to the inability of the proximal tubules to reabsorb all of the filtered glucose. Blood glucose is generally unaffected.

C. Fanconi syndrome is not likely to be associated with an elevated BUN and creatinine. Other features of Fanconi syndrome include glycosuria and aminoaciduria. The syndrome consists of generalized proximal tubular dysfunction with decreased reabsorption of glucose, phosphorus, amino acids, and bicarbonate. Potassium wasting is also a common feature. In the first year of life, Fanconi syndrome is secondary to cystinosis (lysosomal cystine storage) until proven otherwise.

D. In proximal tubular acidosis, the kidneys can produce acid urine because the problem is in reabsorption of bicarbonate. When acidosis exists, the decreased filtered bicarbonate can all be reabsorbed, resulting in little distal delivery of bicarbonate. The distal tubular acidification can then function normally. Urine is considered "acid" when pH is *below* 6.0.

E. Hypophosphatemic rickets can be the consequence of Fanconi syndrome, especially when it is due to cystinosis. This rickets is generally not associated with hypocalcemia, and therefore PTH is unaffected.

87. **C.** Patients who take OCPs have a reduced risk of ovarian cancer that occurs after relatively short-term use (5 years) and persists for 10 to 20 years after their use has been discontinued.

A, B, D. Benefits of OCPs include a decreased incidence of anemia due to reduction of blood loss at each menses, an improvement in acne due to a decrease in free testosterone, and a reduced risk of endometrial cancer.

E. OCPs can cause venous thromboembolism, resulting in stroke and pulmonary embolus.

88. **A.** In Duchenne muscular dystrophy, the calf muscles may feel rubbery and appear enlarged.

B. While some head control problems may be detected early, the hip-girdle weakness does not appear until the second or third year. Pelvic weakness is detected by a waddling gait, wide-based stance, and a Gower sign (propping hands on thighs to push up to a standing position).

C. The CK level is extremely high, even in the earliest stages of the disease.

D. The disease is X-linked and is found in about 1 in 3600 boys.

E. The muscle degeneration seen with Duchenne muscular dystrophy is a painless process that is not associated with muscle spasm or myalgias. The muscle biopsy shows atrophic and hypertrophic muscle fibers and immunohistochemical staining shows deficient or defective dystrophin. Cardiomyopathy is a constant feature of this disease and repeated cardiac assessment is indicated. Death occurs by age 18, usually due to pneumonia, respiratory failure, or heart failure.

89. **D.** Nephropathy secondary to vesicoureteral reflux is one of the most common causes of hypertension in children.

A. Even the first documented UTI in a boy should be investigated to rule out significant urologic abnormalities. Generally, renal ultrasound and voiding cystogram are indicated. The first UTI in a girl under 4 to 5 years of age should also be investigated further.

B. Significant vesicoureteral reflux has been associated with urinary tract infection. However, it is generally felt that the reflux is more causative, and that *significant* reflux does not result from urinary tract infection. The more severe grades of reflux (grade 3 to 5) are more often associated with urinary tract infection and/or reflux nephropathy.

C. Untreated significant vesicoureteral reflux has been associated with end-stage renal disease. It has accounted for 15% to 20% of end-stage kidney disease in the past before greater attention had been placed on the management of UTIs and reflux. End-stage disease is less common now in children followed and treated appropriately.

E. Indeed, vesicoureteral reflux is an inherited trait. While the incidence is as high as 30% to 35% in siblings, most are asymptomatic. About 12% of asymptomatic siblings with reflux have evidence of renal scarring.

90. **A.** Secondary bacterial infection is a common complication of atopic dermatitis and often results from poorly controlled disease and/or pruritis. Antihistamines should be used as an adjunct to control pruritis, while oral antibiotics, such as cephalexin, are used to treat the concurrent infection.

B. Short baths with tepid water are recommended for patients with atopic dermatitis. Excessively warm baths or longer baths will further dry the skin and exacerbate the underlying affected skin.

C. Steroid creams used to treat and control the patchy, erythematous skin of atopic dermatitis need to be applied before an emollient.

D. Cooler, humid ambient temperatures will have less of an effect on drying out the skin than warmer, more arid temperatures.

E. Lubrication needs to be used liberally and almost cannot be too liberal.

91. **B.** Growth delay is a characteristic of uremia secondary to poor response to growth hormone. Other factors include poor nutrition, acidosis, and renal osteodystrophy. Bone age is therefore generally delayed.

A. Anemia in chronic renal failure is usually normocytic, and is secondary to deficiency of erythropoietin production in the kidneys.

C. Osteopenia, not osteosclerosis, would be expected. Rickets is a part of the osteodystrophy of chronic renal disease. It is due to the decreased production of 1,20-dihydrocholecalciferol, the active metabolite of vitamin D. The secondary effects of this deficiency are decreased intestinal absorption of calcium, and failure in calcification of the osteoid to form new bone.

D. Hyperparathyroidism, not hypoparathyroidism, in chronic renal failure results from the lack of vitamin D, poor absorption of calcium, and phosphorus retention—all of which stimulate the parathyroid glands.

E. Most often, the urine in patients with chronic renal failure is closer to isotonic with osmolality near 300, and specific gravity near 1.010. There is usually a concentrating defect.

92. **D.** Vulvovaginal candidiasis causes a discharge that is classically thick, white, cottage cheese-like, and adherent to the vaginal walls. The discharge usually has no odor. The vaginal pH is normally less than 4.5 and is unchanged with a candidal infection. KOH prep is helpful with visualizing the yeast and pseudohyphae by lysing the epithelial cells. Oral fluconazole offers a single-dose treatment.

A. Sitz baths may provide some comfort but will not treat the underlying infection.

B. Topical azole creams can be used but length of therapy is 7 days and compliance may serve as a barrier in the adolescent population.

C. Azithromycin as a single dose would be acceptable for the treatment of *Chlamydia trachomatis*.

E. Metronidazole would be used to treat bacterial vaginosis.

93. **A.** Diabetes type I and other autoimmune diseases such as rheumatoid arthritis, thyroid disease, and IgA deficiency are indeed associated with celiac, another autoimmune disease. In those with celiac disease an autoimmune process takes place after exposure to the protein gluten. This protein is found in wheat, rye, and barley. Normally not the targets of the immune system, portions of this protein are attacked as well as some other human proteins. The immune response leads to inflammation and ultimately damage to the local area.

B. Those with strict adherence to a gluten-free diet will have fewer complications, including a reduced chance of GI malignancy.

C. Polycythemia, or an elevated hematocrit, is not associated with celiac disease. In fact, the opposite is true and anemia is very frequently associated with celiac disease, with the disruption of iron and vitamin B12 absorption.

D. Cleaning solutions are not associated with celiac disease.

E. Decreased albumin is another factor pointing to the ongoing malabsorption that takes place in celiac disease.

94. **B.** The conjunctival injection with Kawasaki disease is nonexudative and typically involves the bulbar conjunctiva. To meet the criteria for classic Kawasaki disease, there should be evidence of fever for at least 5 days plus four of the following five criteria: 1) bulbar conjunctival injection without exudates, 2) mucosal changes such as dry, fissured lips; strawberry tongue or injected pharynx, 3) unilateral cervical lymphadenopathy greater than 1.5 cm usually, 4) induration or edema of the hands and feet, and 5) generalized erythematous rash, which can vary from maculopapular to one resembling erythema multiforme. Five days of fever, three of the above criteria, plus coronary artery abnormalities will also confirm the diagnosis of classic Kawasaki disease.

A. Cervical lymphadenopathy greater than 1.5 cm is one of the criteria associated with the diagnosis of Kawasaki disease.

C. Oral ulcerations are a clinical criteria associated with systemic lupus erythematous.

D. Mitral valve regurgitation is often seen with rheumatic heart disease. Active carditis is one of the major Jones criteria used to make the diagnosis of rheumatic fever. (See the explanation to question 22 for a listing of the Jones criteria.)

E. Scrotal edema can be seen in Kawasaki disease secondary to an associated hypoalbuminemia that may occur. It is not a clinical criteria used in making the diagnosis of Kawasaki disease. Patients with Henoch-Schönlein purpura (HSP) are often noted to have scrotal edema on exam as well.

95. **D.** The symptoms described of chest discomfort, palpitations, near syncope, and dyspnea, in an otherwise healthy patient, are worrisome for serious cardiac and/or pulmonary problems and need immediate evaluation. Although the scenario offers the choice to call the parents to pick up their son, ambulatory transport to an ER would be recommended if the symptoms are severe or persistent.

A. It would not be appropriate to try albuterol, as this may have unwanted side effects such as tachycardia.

B. Placing the patient supine with elevated legs for 15 minutes without any further medical attention would not be appropriate.

C. Waiting a week for further evaluation given the acute nature of the symptoms would be wholly inappropriate.

E. Although taking the patient's pulse during another episode may be helpful, future diagnostic evaluation is needed to prevent or establish the etiology for his symptoms.

96. **B.** This particular exam and symptoms point to the diagnosis of hypertrophic cardiomyopathy. The murmur is typically heard at the lower left sternal border as a systolic ejection grade II-IV/VI murmur. The murmur would be expected to decrease with valsalva maneuvers, such as squatting, and increase with standing. Sharp upstroke of brachial pulses is characteristic. ECG findings of left ventricular hypertrophy would be expected, as would deep Q waves in leads V5 and V6.

A, E. Digitalis and other drugs, such as albuterol, may increase the tone of the heart, resulting in negative effects which can worsen the degree of obstruction.

C. A heart rate of 100 would not be consistent with SVT.

D. There is nothing to suggest dextrocardia in this case.

97. **E.** Lactase deficiency or lactose intolerance is a very common problem in the United States. The intolerance can be partial to complete and can be associated with other disease processes. There is a breath hydrogen study available for further confirmation.

A. Treatment for partial intolerance may be to restrict lactose until asymptomatic.

B. Those of European descent are affected the least, while those of Asian descent are affected the most. African-Americans are very commonly affected.

C. The problem occurs when increased lactose is presented to intestinal bacteria and an osmotic diarrhea ensues.

D. If milk products are reduced significantly then calcium supplements are indicated.

98. **C.** All of the answers listed—congenital hypothyroidism, duodenal atresia, Hirschsprung disease, Meckel diverticulum, and TEF—are associated with trisomy 21 (Down syndrome). Hirschsprung disease should be considered whenever there has been no passage of meconium in the first 48 hours. In Hirschsprung disease, there is an absence of ganglionic cells in the bowel wall, confirmed by biopsy. The result is delayed passage of meconium or further problems with chronic constipation.

A. Hypothyroidism will cause constipation in time.

B. Duodenal atresia should cause upper GI tract symptoms such as early emesis.

D. Meckel diverticulum should not delay the stooling, and would be expected to present with hematochezia.

E. TEFs do not delay passage of stool and often present with choking during feeds and/or excessive secretions.

99. **B. The child has amblyopia of the left eye.** Early diagnosis and treatment are crucial to this disease. Amblyopia is characterized by central suppression of the vision of one or both eyes. In a literate child, the best corrected vision of 20/30 or worse in one *or both* eyes, not explained by eye pathology, is diagnostic. Correcting the vision with the appropriate glasses, and occluding or blurring the vision of the better-seeing eye to eliminate suppression of the affected eye, are key therapeutic elements.

A, C. Therapy initiated in teenage years will not typically be successful, and initiating therapy prior to age 8 is best.

D. Patching the left eye is not appropriate, as the child has amblyopia of the left eye.

E. Simply realigning the eye will not force the brain to stop suppressing the eye, so surgery is often deferred until the amblyopia is resolved.

100. **C. There are several items to ensure in follow-up evaluations of amblyopia.** Assessing degree of vision improvement, and ensuring that the dominant eye has not been weakened, are both critical. Encouragement of the patient and family during this tiresome and stigmatizing treatment is needed. Subsequent exams are scheduled weeks or months apart, depending on the age of the child. The plasticity of the visual system demands that younger children be reevaluated at intervals no more than 1 week for each month of their age (a 4-month-old should be reassessed no later than 4 weeks after therapy is initiated.). The typical interval for older children is 3 months.

A, B, D. These follow-up times are incorrect. See explanation for C.

E. Follow-up of patients with ambylopia is critical. See explanation for C.

Setting 3: Inpatient Facilities

You have general admitting privileges to the hospital. You may see patients in
the critical care unit, the pediatrics unit, the maternity unit, or recovery room.
You may also be called to see patients in the psychiatric unit. A short-stay unit
serves patients who are undergoing same-day operations or who are being
held for observation. There are adjacent nursing home/extended-care facilities
and a detoxification unit where you may see patients.

101. A term infant is born to a mother whose perinatal labs include HIV nonreactive; RPR− (rapid plasma reagin−); GBS− (group B streptococcus−); hepatitis B−; blood type, O+. The infant is approximately 20 hours old and appears to be jaundiced to the chest. He is exclusively breastfed and clinically has been doing well. The most likely cause of his jaundice is:

A. Breastfeeding jaundice
B. Breastmilk jaundice
C. Biliary atresia
D. ABO incompatibility
E. Physiologic jaundice

102. During an initial newborn exam you detect a palpable clunk in the patient's left hip during your Ortolani and Barlow maneuvers. You are concerned for developmental dysplasia of the hip (DDH). Your next course of action would be:

A. Obtain radiographs of the pelvis and hips
B. Obtain hip ultrasound
C. Place the infant in triple diapers
D. Orthopedic referral
E. Observe and follow-up in 1 month

103. A 6-year-old boy is admitted with a 1-month history of cervical lymphadenitis that has continued to progress despite outpatient treatment with amoxicillin-clavulanate (Augmentin). The child has been clinically well without any other constitutional symptoms. A previously placed PPD measures 5 mm. His physical exam is pertinent for right cervical lymphadenopathy measuring about 3 to 4 cm with some overlying tenderness and erythema. A needle biopsy of the lymph node is undertaken (Figure 103). The most appropriate management of this patient would be:

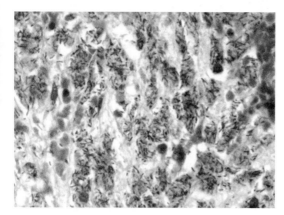

Figure 103 • Image courtesy of the Department of Pathology, Phoenix Children's Hospital, Phoenix, Arizona.

A. Surgical excision of the lymph node
B. IV therapy with ampicillin-sulbactam (Unasyn)
C. Referral to an oncologist
D. Intralesional injection of corticosteroids
E. IV therapy with ceftazidime and gentamycin

104. A 2-week-old infant is admitted to the wards with a 3-day history of poor feeding, tachypnea, and vomiting. Her perinatal history is unremarkable. Vitals are T, 37.6°C; P, 150; R, 52; and BP, 80/55, with a physical exam that is remarkable for a slightly sunken anterior fontanelle, tachypnea with clear breath sounds, and mottled skin appearance. Labs obtained in the ER show a normal CBC and differential; Na^+, 135; K^+, 2.6; Cl^-, 89; CO_2, 7; BUN, 16; and creatinine, 0.5. Which of the following would be the most useful step in arriving at a final diagnosis?

A. Obtaining an ammonia level
B. Completing a full septic evaluation
C. Urine for organic acids
D. 17-OH-progesterone
E. TSH

105. You are called to the bedside of a 5-day-old preterm infant for increasing respiratory distress. The infant has been on a ventilator since birth. The physical exam is significant for tachypnea, retractions, and some decreased breath sounds noted on the right. You request a STAT x-ray (Figure 105). The next most appropriate step in management is:

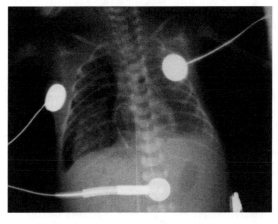

Figure 105 • Image courtesy of the Department of Radiology, Phoenix Children's Hospital, Phoenix, Arizona.

A. Immediate broad-spectrum antibiotics
B. Confirmatory left lateral decubitus radiograph
C. Placement of a chest tube
D. Confirmatory ultrasound or CT
E. Immediate albuterol treatment

106. The housestaff presents a case of a 13-year-old female with chronic abdominal cramping to their attending physician. Their thorough history and physical exam demonstrates a Tanner stage 2 female with flattening of the growth curve over the last 2 years and a right lower quadrant mass. In discussing the differential diagnosis of these problems, a senior resident states that inflammatory bowel disease is high on the list. A discussion then ensues about the differences between Crohn disease and ulcerative colitis. Which of the following statements would be most accurate to share with the patient and her family?

- **A.** Extra-intestinal manifestations occur in both diseases, and include problems such as peripheral arthritis, erythema nodosum, and anemia
- **B.** Colectomy is advised in all patients with ulcerative colitis within 2 years of diagnosis
- **C.** Ulcerative colitis patients typically have more difficulty with fissures and fistulas
- **D.** Skip lesions are required for the diagnosis of Crohn, but are common in ulcerative colitis as well
- **E.** Esophageal and stomach involvement is quite rare in Crohn and if found would suggest eosinophilic gastroenteritis as a comorbid condition

107. A 15-year-old male with Burkitt lymphoma in remission is transferred to the PICU with active seizures. The patient is currently taking antibiotics for pneumonia. His physical exam is nonfocal and the patient does not appear to be dehydrated. Serum electrolytes reveal a serum sodium of 112 mEq/L. What would be the most appropriate action at this time?

- **A.** Infusion of 3% hypertonic saline to acutely raise the serum sodium to 120 to 125 mEq/L
- **B.** Furosemide (Lasix) at 1 mg/kg IV
- **C.** Fluid restriction to 80% maintenance fluid
- **D.** Acute correction of serum sodium to 140 mEq/L
- **E.** Phosphenytoin 18 mg/kg IV load

108. A 4-week-old ex-34-week preemie is admitted with retractions, tachypnea, and an oxygen saturation of 80% on room air. The respiratory rate is 70 breaths/min and wheezes are heard diffusely in all lung fields. A nasal-pharyngeal wash demonstrates the presence of respiratory syncytial virus (RSV). The parents ask you what you can do in the PICU to help their child and relieve his respiratory distress. You respond:

- **A.** Steroids can be administered but will take 6 to 12 hours before we begin to see an effect
- **B.** Supportive care is the mainstay of bronchiolitis therapy
- **C.** Antibiotics may be administered to prevent impending respiratory failure
- **D.** An infusion of RSV intravenous immunoglobulin (IVIG) will hasten the patient's recovery from bronchiolitis
- **E.** Continuous high-dose bronchodilator therapy should relieve this patient's respiratory distress

109. A 3-year-old boy has been admitted to the hospital with a history of fever, severe abdominal pain, and diarrhea. An outside CT scan of his abdomen was obtained and read as normal except for a thickening and inflammation of the pancreatic head. Further laboratory evaluation reveals an amylase of 1900 U/L and a lipase of 5000 U/L. Which of the following is an accurate statement regarding this patient's condition?

A. Blunt trauma is a common etiology
B. Amylase is always abnormal at presentation
C. Elevated amylase levels are usually diagnostic
D. Ranson's criteria can be used to predict prognosis
E. Pseudocyst development is a common complication

110. A child presents on the hospital ward with respiratory distress, exhibited by nasal flaring, intercostal retractions, grunting respirations, and cyanosis. You start oxygen by facemask, but the child is still in significant respiratory distress and becomes apneic. The best next step is:

A. Start chest compressions
B. Perform a Heimlich maneuver, as the child may have aspirated something
C. Obtain a blood gas
D. Send the child to the radiology department for a chest x-ray
E. Start bag-valve-mask ventilations with 100% oxygen

111. A newborn is found on initial exam to have a 2-cm round mass over the nasal bridge. It is soft to touch, slightly bluish in color, and darkens and swells slightly when the baby cries. An exam light transilluminates the lesion. The best next step in the management of this finding is:

A. Reassure the parents it will resolve with time
B. Obtain a biopsy
C. Inject the lesion with steroid to induce involution
D. Massage the lesion or apply a pressure bandage to induce microembolization
E. Order an MRI of the baby's head

112. A 2-year-old boy is admitted to the hospital with high fever for 5 or 6 days, swelling of the hands and feet, scarletiniform changes of the tongue, a generalized red maculopapular rash, dry red cracked lips, and scleral injection. The toddler looks miserable out of proportion to his physical findings. His initial lab work-up reveals an erythrocyte sedimentation rate (ESR) greater than 100 and thrombocytosis with a platelet count of 60,000. Which of the following is the best initial treatment?

A. Cardiac catheterization and long-term follow-up by cardiology
B. IVIG 2 g/kg IV and high-dose aspirin orally
C. Aspirin 5 mg/kg by mouth (PO) daily
D. Steroid therapy
E. Avoid influenza and varicella vaccines until the child is better

---

The next 2 questions (items 113-114) correspond to the following vignette.

An 18-month-old girl is admitted from the ED with a chief complaint of a draining sore on her right buttock. Her grandmother reports that she first noticed an area of redness on the child's right buttock 5 days ago. Over this time period, the area enlarged and became tender and warm. Yesterday it spontaneously opened and started draining a yellow-red discharge. On physical exam, the toddler is alert and prefers to lie on her side because of the pain. Her vital signs reveal a temperature of 38.6°C and a pulse of 130. Blood pressure and respiratory rate are normal. The rest of the exam is normal except for the right buttock. There is a 6-cm area of erythema and a central 2-cm area of induration. In the center of this indurated area is a small opening through which you see the yellow-red discharge seeping out.

113. The most likely diagnosis is:

   A. Osteomyelitis of the sacrum
   B. Perirectal abscess
   C. Irritant contact dermatitis
   D. Candidal dermatitis
   E. Crohn disease

114. The most appropriate next step in management would be:

   A. Surgical consult for incision and drainage
   B. Primary closure of the draining site with sutures
   C. Oral amoxicillin for 10 days
   D. Sterile dressing application and follow-up with PCP in 1 week
   E. Barium enema

End of set

---

115. A 3300-g newborn male is born at 39 weeks gestational age to a 25-year-old mother. Prenatal labs show that the mother is rubella immune, RPR nonreactive, HIV nonreactive, hepatitis B negative, but GBS positive. The mother received IV ampicillin in adequate doses more than 4 hours before delivery. On initial exam, the baby's vital signs and physical exam are normal. He is voiding and stooling well and breastfeeding without difficulties. The most appropriate next step in management would be:

   A. Lumbar puncture (LP)
   B. Chest x-ray
   C. Observation for 48 hours
   D. CBC and blood culture
   E. Empiric IV antibiotics for 72 hours

116. You are following a 2-year-old boy with septo-optic dysplasia (SOD) in the hospital for viral gastroenteritis and dehydration. Which medication needs to be adjusted during this hospitalization and illness?

    A. Thyroid supplementation
    B. Insulin
    C. Glucocorticoid supplementation
    D. Vasopressin (DDAVP)
    E. Growth hormone (GH)

117. You are attending the delivery of a term infant who was born via normal spontaneous vaginal delivery with thick meconium. The baby is suctioned at the perineum and then handed to you. You notice slow irregular respirations, a heart rate of 130, limp muscle tone, grimacing, and a pale blue body throughout. What would this infant's Apgar score be at 1 minute if the exam remains unchanged?

    A. 0
    B. 2
    C. 4
    D. 5
    E. 8
    F. 12

118. A $2^1/_2$-week-old infant presents with a 4-day history of vomiting, decreased intake, and lethargy. The physical exam is significant for a mildly sunken fontanelle, dry mouth, and decreased activity. You notice that the scrotal sacs are hyperpigmented and small. The testes are nonpalpable and there is mild hypospadias. Electrolytes are obtained and show Na^+, 125 mmol/L; K^+, 6.4 mmol/L; Cl^-, 103 mmol/L; CO_2, 15 mmol/L; and glucose, 50 mg/dL. Which of the following is accurate information to give to the family regarding this patient's illness?

    A. This condition is inherited as an autosomal dominant trait
    B. The most common form of the disease is 11-hydroxylase deficiency
    C. Treatment includes replacement of cortisol and aldosterone
    D. Ultrasound is indicated to localize the testes
    E. Laboratory evaluation should include AM serum cortisol levels

119. In the delivery room, you notice that a newborn infant already has two teeth present in the lower gum. The pregnancy was uneventful without any infections and the mother received no medications other than prenatal vitamins. Which of the following is appropriate information to tell this infant's mother?

    A. A deep root system is typically developed
    B. Natal teeth are most commonly found in the position of the maxillary central incisors
    C. A family history of natal teeth is common
    D. There is no risk of aspiration
    E. There is no association with cleft palate

120. A 10-month-old baby is noted to be chronically irritable. His mother, who wears a veil and gown and is a vegetarian for religious reasons, has been breastfeeding the baby exclusively. The baby's fontanelle is still open and is noted to be bulging. On physical exam you find frontal bossing, widening of the wrists, and bowed legs. Because of the irritability and bulging fontanelle, you order an MRI scan. It is reported as normal aside from showing evidence of increased intracranial pressure. An LP yields normal cerebrospinal fluid and an elevated opening pressure. The next step in the management of this patient would be to:

A. Perform serial LPs
B. Prescribe acetazolamide (Diamox)
C. Administer corticosteroids
D. Prescribe vitamin D and calcium supplements
E. Refer patient to a neurosurgeon

121. A baby seen in the newborn nursery is found to have a loud heart murmur. The baby has been feeding poorly. The chest radiograph demonstrates decreased pulmonary vascular flow and you are considering tricuspid atresia as a possible diagnosis. In preparing to tell the parents about their baby's heart defect, which of the following is most accurate?

A. In this condition, blood cannot flow from the right atrium to the right ventricle
B. In most cases, a patent ductus arteriosus (PDA) allows blood to get to the lungs
C. Most patients do not have cyanosis in the newborn period
D. The cardiogram generally shows right ventricular hypertrophy
E. The goal of medical and surgical treatment is to decrease blood flow to the lungs

122. A 3-day-old preterm infant develops intermittent apnea spells lasting greater than 20 seconds, accompanied by bradycardia. Investigation reveals no apparent infection or metabolic imbalance. These episodes seem to respond to gentle cutaneous stimulation. Which one of the following would be true for the management of this baby?

A. The baby is too young to consider this idiopathic apnea
B. No medication has been shown to be beneficial for frequent apnea
C. Correction of anemia would have no effect on the frequency of apnea
D. If the episodes are frequent, nasal continuous positive airway pressure (CPAP) might be beneficial
E. Apnea of prematurity usually resolves at 2 months of age

123. A 4-year-old boy is seen because of increased thirst and increased urination. He was toilet trained at 2 years, but he still wets the bed every night. Your concern is that this boy could have diabetes insipidus (DI) or psychogenic water drinking. A morning urine specimen after an 8-hour fast shows a specific gravity of 1.005. His serum sodium is 140 mEq/L. What would be your next step?

A. Administer vasopressin to see whether his urine can concentrate
B. Administer a sodium load to see whether his kidneys can respond by increasing sodium excretion
C. Increase the overnight fasting test to 12 to 15 hours to see whether his urine can concentrate
D. Perform a daytime water deprivation test, measuring any changes in urine concentration and serum osmolality
E. Because his serum sodium is normal, advise the parents that there is no need for further tests

124. An infant is born with port-wine nevus distributed and well-demarcated over the distribution of the right trigeminal area of the face. Which one of the following may apply to this syndrome?

    A. Pulsed dye laser treatments are frequently used and are quite effective for the skin lesions

    B. While seizures are common, most patients can be readily controlled with anticonvulsant therapy

    C. Medical management is the only avenue for the treatment of recalcitrant seizures

    D. Glaucoma on the affected side is always apparent in the first month of life

    E. Subsequent siblings have a 25% risk of being affected because this condition is autosomal recessive

125. You are called by the nurse to evaluate a term 3-hour-old infant who was born to a 25-year-old mother with unremarkable prenatal labs and an uncomplicated pregnancy. The baby was born via scheduled cesarean section without previous rupture of membranes secondary to a previous child born via cesarean section. On physical exam you notice a mild to moderately tachypneic infant with some coarse breath sounds bilaterally and mild intercostal retractions; the remainder of the physical exam is normal. The child is saturating 98% on room air. A chest radiograph is obtained (Figure 125). Your next step in management would be:

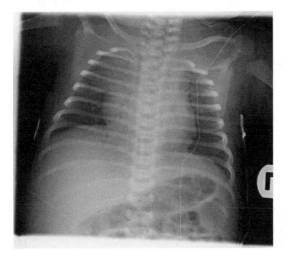

Figure 125 • Image courtesy of the Department of Radiology, Phoenix Children's Hospital, Phoenix, Arizona.

    A. Place the infant on supplemental oxygen

    B. Immediately administer antibiotics

    C. Draw a CBC/blood culture and then administer antibiotics

    D. Perform an ECHO

    E. Careful observation only

126. A 7-year-old African-American girl is admitted to the hospital for the evaluation of fever with a limp. Her father has noticed low-grade fevers intermittently for the past 4 weeks. Over this time period, the girl has had progressive pain in the right knee and is now refusing to walk or bear weight on that leg. She does have sickle cell disease. On physical exam, she is febrile and irritable. The right knee is slightly swollen compared to the left. She refuses to stand unassisted. Her total serum white blood cell count and ESR are elevated. Plain radiographs of the right lower extremity reveal periosteal elevation and subperiosteal fluid collection of the medial, distal right femur. The most likely causative bacterial pathogen for this child's illness is:

A. *Pseudomonas aeruginosa*
B. *Salmonella*
C. *Brucella*
D. *Staphylococcus aureus*
E. *Candida albicans*

127. A 6-month-old child is in the PICU with pneumococcal meningitis. He weighs 5 kg. He initially presented 2 days ago. Over the last 24 hours he has received D5 0.2% normal saline IV at 20 mL/hr. Electrolytes reveal a serum sodium of 123 mEq/L, potassium of 4.5 mEq/L, chloride of 90 mEq/L, and serum CO_2 of 23 mEq/L. Heart rate is 140 beats/min, respiratory rate is 30 breaths/min, and blood pressure is 110/70 mm Hg. Urine output has been 0.8 mL/kg/hr. Urine osmolality is 800 mEq/L. What would be the best way to initially begin to correct this serum sodium?

A. Add sodium to the child's formula
B. Change the IV fluid to 0.5 normal saline
C. Fluid restriction to insensible losses
D. Administer a thiazide diuretic
E. Give 20 mL/kg normal saline bolus over 10 minutes or less

128. You are called emergently to the bedside of a 9-month-old child who appears to have stopped breathing. On your physical exam you note no active respirations and no audible heartbeat or palpable pulses. After establishment of the airway, chest compressions are best performed on an infant by:

A. Using the heel of one hand
B. Using two fingers depressing the lower half of the sternum
C. Depressing the sternum 1.5 to 2 inches
D. Depressing the chest at a rate of 90 to 100 times per minute
E. Depressing the sternum less than one third of the depth of the chest

129. A child with acute lymphoblastic leukemia has a central line placed for ease of administration of medications and blood products. His induction chemotherapy includes dexamethasone, vincristine, and asparaginase. He is in remission 7 days after the start of therapy. After 2 weeks of therapy, he develops swelling of his chest wall on the side of the central line. On physical exam, venous distention is noted around the area of swelling. His most likely diagnosis is:

A. Cellulitis of his chest wall
B. Abscess of deep structures of the chest
C. Leukemic infiltration of his skin
D. Deep venous thrombosis of his subclavian vein
E. Osteomyelitis of his ribs

130. A 14-year-old boy is hospitalized with intractable seizures of unknown cause lasting several hours. His condition was stabilized after the first 6 hours in the hospital. His vital signs are relatively normal, and his seizures are controlled. However, his urine has become brown in color, and he is becoming progressively more oliguric. Exam of the urine shows a 2+ reaction for protein, 4+ hematest, specific gravity 1.025, pH 5.5, and surprisingly few RBCs. Electrolytes reveal a mild metabolic acidosis, and are otherwise normal. His serum phosphorus is 9.0 mg/dL, calcium 8.0 mg/dL, BUN 15 mg/dL, and creatinine 0.6 mg/dL. Your immediate next course of treatment would be which one of the following:

A. Administer an intravenous bolus of normal saline 20 mL/kg, followed by maintenance-type fluids
B. Withhold IV fluids and administer furosemide IV 2 mg/kg
C. Administer a 20 mL/kg bolus of normal saline followed by mannitol 0.5 g/kg over 30 minutes, then continue with a sodium bicarbonate solution to maintain his urine pH near 7.5, watching his serum chemistries for evidence of renal failure
D. Begin maintenance fluids at a volume equal to insensible water losses plus urine output, awaiting the need to institute dialysis
E. Begin dialysis, anticipating that he will develop renal failure

131. An 8-year-old boy, who has been developmentally normal, has started to have some gait disturbance and developmental regression. His speech has become slurred, and there is a slight hand tremor bilaterally. His muscles seem tight, and there is some ataxia. Some dysarthria is also noted. Basic chemistries reveal serum sodium of 128 mEq/L, potassium 5.4 mEq/L, chloride 106 mEq/L, and CO_2 20 mEq/L. You suspect that this boy has some sort of neurodegenerative disorder. Which one of the following statements regarding neurodegenerative disorders is true?

A. Most neurodegenerative disorders are sporadic and not hereditary
B. The metabolic defect in most neurodegenerative disorders is unknown
C. Adrenal insufficiency should be a consideration in this patient
D. Adrenoleukodystrophy and metachromatic leukodystrophy are variants of the same disease
E. All the sphingolipidoses involve the storage of an abnormal lipid

132. A 3-month-old male infant is hospitalized with nonsupperative indolent infections of the skin and mouth. He also has had diarrhea for the past 4 weeks, failure to thrive, and a rather persistent respiratory infection. He was delivered at term without complications. Further pertinent history reveals that his umbilical cord did not separate until 6 weeks of age. Which one of the following tests would most likely confirm a diagnosis?

A. Test for quantitative serum immunoglobulin level
B. Test for serum complement deficiency
C. Test for leukocyte killing deficiency
D. Test for leukocyte chemotaxis
E. Test for leukocyte adhesion deficiency

133. A 3-month-old boy who was born with a large abdomen presents to the clinic. The pregnancy was characterized by oligohydramnios. The infant developed respiratory distress soon after birth, and required a ventilator for several days. There are large palpable masses bilaterally. Abdominal ultrasound shows enlarged bilateral renal masses, which are echo dense with obscured corticomedullary junctions. Serum chemistries are normal. The BUN is 10 mg/dL and the creatinine 0.5 mg/dL. A renal biopsy is performed (Figure 133). Counseling the parents about this child's illness would include which of the following?

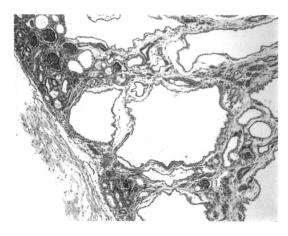

Figure 133 • Image courtesy of the Department of Pathology, Phoenix Children's Hospital, Phoenix, Arizona.

A. This is an X-linked recessive disorder
B. Renal failure usually will not develop until he is an adult
C. Fifty percent of subsequent children, both male and female, will be affected
D. Large cysts of varying sizes are present early in this condition
E. Hepatic fibrosis is a common feature of this disorder

134. A newborn infant is noted to have dysmorphic features in the delivery room. The significant physical findings include hypotonia, microcephaly, wide-spaced first and second toes, simian crease, and epicanthal folds. Counseling the parents about this newborn should include:

A. Cardiac defects are seen in about 60%
B. Sterility is nearly universal in males
C. Mental retardation occurs in nearly all patients
D. Gastroschisis is commonly associated with this condition
E. Cardiac defects are seen in about 60%, and sterility is nearly universal in males
F. Cardiac defects are seen in about 60%, sterility is nearly universal in males, and mental retardation occurs in nearly all patients
G. Cardiac defects are seen in about 60%, sterility is nearly universal in males, mental retardation occurs in nearly all patients, and gastroschisis is commonly associated with this condition

135. A 4-year-old boy with known insulin-dependent diabetes is admitted to the hospital with significant lab values as follows: glucose, 650; sodium, 130; potassium, 2.5; chloride, 89; CO_2, 8; BUN, 29; and creatinine, 0.9. His physical exam is significant for dry, cracked mucous membranes, and a capillary refill of 4 seconds. Which of the following is considered to be a standard component of first-line medical therapy in this patient?

A. Administration of insulin by IV bolus
B. Administration of long-acting insulin subcutaneously
C. Administration of IV sodium bicarbonate
D. Parenteral rehydration
E. Administration of IM glucagon

136. You are called to examine a newborn infant with tachypnea. The infant's mother received no prenatal care. Vital signs are T, 37.6°C; P, 170; R, 75; BP 85/50; and saturations of 80% on room air with a physical exam significant for clear lung sounds with obvious tachypnea and no audible murmur with a normal S1 and single loud S2. A chest x-ray shows increased pulmonary markings with an egg-shaped cardiac silhouette. Which of the following would be most beneficial in the management of this infant?

A. Indomethacin
B. Captopril
C. Surfactant
D. Prostaglandin E_1
E. Propranolol

137. A 10-year-old girl who has lost significant weight over the past year is admitted to the hospital. She has been having gradually increasing difficulty swallowing solid foods, but she has been able to hold down liquids fairly well. There has been occasional vomiting, but no history of aspiration pneumonia. Her barium esophagram is shown (Figure 137). The most likely diagnosis is:

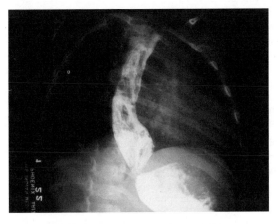

Figure 137 • Image courtesy of the Department of Radiology, Phoenix Children's Hospital, Phoenix, Arizona.

A. Hiatal hernia
B. Achalasia
C. Gastroesophageal reflux (GER)
D. Pyloric stenosis
E. Esophageal burn from caustic ingestion

138. You are admitting an 18-month-old toddler from the ED with rotavirus-positive acute gastroenteritis. She has been fluid resuscitated in the ED and is now rehydrated on physical exam. Even though maintenance IV fluids are running, she continues with frequent loose stools, but is not vomiting and acts hungry. The nurse is asking you what diet should be ordered. The most appropriate diet for this child would be:

A. NPO (nothing by mouth, IVF only)
B. BRAT diet (bananas, rice, applesauce, and toast)
C. Age-appropriate diet
D. Clear liquids only
E. Thick liquids only

139. You are called to see a newborn infant in the hospital because of feeding difficulties. The nurse reports that the child appears to be gagging with feedings and has excessive saliva. You attempt to pass an NG tube, which is unsuccessful. Which of the following is most accurate in reference to this infant's problem?

A. The least common form has the esophagus ending in a blind pouch with a distal connection between the trachea and esophagus
B. Ten percent of patients have associated anomalies such as VATER/VACTERL syndromes
C. H-type fistulas may not be detected until later in life
D. H-type fistulas are the most common type
E. Aspiration is infrequent with tracheoesophageal fistulas (TEFs)

140. A 2-month-old boy is admitted to the hospital with infantile spasms. His mother is known to have tuberous sclerosis and has normal intelligence. She is concerned that her son may also have tuberous sclerosis. Which of the following is accurate information to give to his mother?

A. Later skin manifestations of tuberous sclerosis may include shagreen patch, subungual fibromas, and café-au-lait spots
B. Mental retardation is not likely because the mother has normal intelligence
C. Tuberous sclerosis rarely affects the kidneys
D. Cataracts are common eye findings in tuberous sclerosis
E. Myxomas of the heart are common in tuberous sclerosis

141. You are called by the nurse to examine a newborn infant because of concerns over a congenital deformity. On the exam of an infant boy you observe a rather severe talipes equinovarus (clubfoot) deformity of the right foot. The parents are visibly upset and have many questions. Which of the following is appropriate information to give them?

A. Positional foot deformity must be treated like a clubfoot deformity
B. Clubfoot deformity has no genetic implications
C. Surgery is usually recommended in the newborn period for moderately severe clubfoot
D. Calf and foot atrophy frequently result in spite of adequate early treatment of clubfoot
E. The deformity in congenital clubfoot is usually limited to the foot and ankle

142. A 10-day-old premature baby in the intensive care nursery develops abdominal distension, bloody stools, and bilious vomiting. The baby has been taking a cow's milk protein-based preterm formula. An abdominal radiograph is obtained (Figure 142). The most appropriate management of this infant would be:

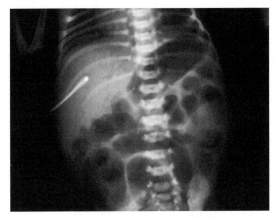

Figure 142 · Image courtesy of the Department of Radiology, Phoenix Children's Hospital, Phoenix, Arizona.

A. Switch to a protein hydrolysate formula
B. No immediate treatment is necessary; repeat radiograph in 24 hours
C. Continue to feed formula; start oral antibiotics
D. Make patient NPO, start IV antibiotics
E. Take patient to OR for bowel resection

143. You are called to the delivery of a full-term infant boy who was found to have the stigmata of Down syndrome. He was born to a 24-year-old primagravida mother with an unremarkable prenatal history. There is no history of the occurrence of Down syndrome in any of the family members on either the father's or the mother's side. Which one of the following statements is true?

A. The likelihood of recurrence in a subsequent offspring is about 1 in 700
B. Only 50% of Down syndrome patients result from trisomy 21
C. Almost all Down syndrome conceptions will carry to term
D. Mosaic Down syndrome results from a meiotic nondisjunction
E. Down syndrome in mothers under 30 years of age is most often a result of trisomy 21

144. You are seeing a newborn term baby in the nursery. All prenatal labs are normal as is the infant's exam. The mother reports that a cousin who visited yesterday has chicken pox. There is a history of varicella in the mother as a child. What would be the next step in the management of this newborn?

A. Acyclovir
B. Varicella-zoster immunoglobulin (VZIG)
C. Observation only
D. Cephazolin
E. Acyclovir and VZIG

145. A newborn is noted to have abdominal distension, vomiting, and failure to pass meconium in the first 48 hours of life. Abdominal radiographs show dilated loops of small bowel with air-fluid levels and a collection of "ground glass" material in the lower abdomen. The surgeon's postoperative diagnosis is meconium ileus. Which of the statements about meconium ileus would be correct information to give to the family?

A. It is commonly seen in Down syndrome
B. About 65% of infants with cystic fibrosis develop meconium ileus
C. It is less common in children whose siblings had meconium ileus
D. Rupture of the bowel wall and peritonitis are not complications of meconium ileus
E. If an enema with a hypertonic solution such as diatrizoate (Gastrografin) does not cause passage of the plug and relief of the obstruction, surgical intervention is necessary

146. A 12-year-old boy with chronic renal failure and a history of noncompliance with dialysis appointments is admitted to the floor. You are called emergently to his bedside by the nurses who fear he is in shock. An electrocardiograph reveals a chaotic rhythm with a widened QRS complex. The most effective management for this child would be:

A. Lidocaine 1 mg/kg IV bolus
B. Calcium chloride (10%), 0.2 mL/kg IV bolus
C. Magnesium sulfate, 25 mg/kg IV bolus
D. Furosemide, 5 mg/kg IV infusion
E. Mannitol, 1 g/kg IV infusion

147. A 4-year-old boy is admitted to the hospital with severe asthma. He has been admitted on two previous occasions. Oxygen saturations are 96% on 2 liters of O_2 by mask. Which one of the following arterial blood gas determinations would suggest this patient should be transferred to the ICU?

A. pH 7.35, HCO_3 20 mEq/L, pCO_2 36 mm Hg
B. pH 7.40, HCO_3 20 mEq/L, pCO_2 32 mm Hg
C. pH 7.40, HCO_3 27 mEq/L, pCO_2 45 mm Hg
D. pH 7.30, HCO_3 17.5 mEq/L, pCO_2 35 mm Hg
E. pH 7.25, HCO_3 13 mEq/L, pCO_2 30 mm Hg

148. A 6-month-old infant hospitalized for diagnostic evaluation of a congenital heart defect has echocardiographic findings consistent with tetralogy of Fallot (overriding aorta, VSD, pulmonary atresia, and right ventricular hypertrophy). You are called to see the child because he has become hypoxic and moderately cyanotic with a bout of crying. What is the first step in managing this "Tet spell"?

A. Reposition the child with knees to chest
B. Administer oxygen
C. Administer an IV fluid bolus
D. Prepare to perform cardiopulmonary resuscitation
E. Administer furosemide

The next 2 questions (items 149-150) correspond to the following vignette.

A 1-week-old baby is admitted from the ED with respiratory distress. Parents report that she has had progressive feeding and breathing difficulties since birth. Now she will only bottle feed small amounts and often will have nonprojectile regurgitation soon after feeding. Her breathing has become more rapid and includes accessory muscle use. On exam, she is afebrile with a respiratory rate of 70. She is mildly dehydrated and acts very hungry. She has mild intercostal retractions and you hear no breath sounds over the left hemithorax. Breath sounds on the right are clear. The rest of the exam is normal. CBC and basic metabolic panel (BMP) from the ED are normal. CXR taken on the way up from the ED is now available for your review (Figure 149).

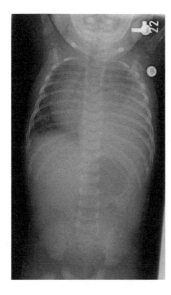

Figure 149 · Image courtesy of the Department of Radiology, Phoenix Children's Hospital, Phoenix, Arizona.

149. The most likely diagnosis is:

    A. Pyloric stenosis
    B. Pneumonia with pleural effusion
    C. TEF
    D. Diaphragmatic hernia
    E. Duodenal atresia

150. The most appropriate next step in management is:

    A. NG tube decompression and surgical consultation
    B. IV antibiotics
    C. Chest tube insertion
    D. Pyloromyotomy
    E. ECHO

End of set

Answer Key

101. D	118. C	135. D
102. D	119. C	136. D
103. A	120. D	137. B
104. C	121. A	138. C
105. C	122. D	139. C
106. A	123. D	140. A
107. A	124. A	141. D
108. B	125. E	142. D
109. A	126. D	143. E
110. E	127. C	144. C
111. E	128. B	145. E
112. B	129. D	146. B
113. B	130. C	147. C
114. A	131. C	148. A
115. C	132. E	149. D
116. C	133. E	150. A
117. C	134. F	

101. **D.** ABO incompatibility most commonly occurs when the mother's blood type is O and the baby is either type A or B. The mother, being type O, has maternal antibodies to both A and B, which results in a hemolytic process that presents as jaundice. A blood type and direct Coombs test should be obtained on all infants born to mothers who are type O.

A. Breastfeeding jaundice typically occurs in the first week of life secondary to a relative state of dehydration as a consequence of decreased breastmilk production.

B. Breastmilk jaundice usually occurs in exclusively breastfed babies in the second to third week of life. It is thought to be related to the intrinsic properties of breastmilk, which may inhibit glucuronyl transferase and the subsequent conjugation of bilirubin.

C. Biliary atresia is a disease that results in varying degrees of malformation to complete absence of the biliary tree. Although a cause of jaundice, biliary atresia typically is detected much later in life with an incidence that approximates 1 in 10,000 to 15,000.

E. By definition, any jaundice within the first 24 hours is pathological and needs further investigation. Physiologic jaundice occurs in term infants on days 2 to 4 and is believed to be related to increased red cell breakdown, increased bilirubin production, and relative immaturity of the liver's conjugation capacity.

102. **D.** If a positive exam is elicited in a newborn, an immediate orthopedic referral is recommended.

A. Radiographs of the pelvis and hips have limited value in the first few months of life when the femoral heads are composed mainly of cartilage. They become more reliable at approximately 4 to 6 months.

B. Although hip ultrasound is a useful exam in evaluating for DDH, treatment decisions are based on the results of the physical exam. A hip ultrasound is not recommended in the newborn with a positive exam.

C. The use of triple diapers is not recommended; they have not been shown to be effective and may even delay the onset of appropriate treatment.

E. An infant with a positive exam and concern for DDH requires fairly urgent, but not emergent, care. Simply observing and following up in 1 month is not acceptable.

103. **A.** The patient has a cervical lymphadenitis caused by atypical mycobacteria. The clinical history of progressing or unimproved cervical lymphadenopathy with minimal to no constitutional symptoms, a weakly positive purified protein derivative (PPD), and the lymph node biopsy showing acid fast bacilli (AFB) confirm the diagnosis. The treatment of choice is complete excision of the lymph node; incomplete excision often results in persistent drainage. Antituberculosis medications are not necessary following excision unless concern for *Myobacteria tuberculosis* cannot be ruled out.

B. IV therapy with ampicillin-sulbactam would be a good choice for the more common bacterial lymphadenitis caused by group A *Streptococcus* or *Staphylococcus aureus*.

C. There are no constitutional symptoms or other physical exam findings to suspect an oncologic process is occurring, so referral is unnecessary.

D. The use of steroids, either intralesional or systemically, is not indicated.

E. Ceftazidime and gentamycin would be appropriate choices for pseudomonal infections.

104. C. The infant in this scenario has a classic presentation of a metabolic disorder with poor feeding and vomiting without any history of fevers. The tachypnea is a result of attempted respiratory compensation for an underlying acidosis. The patient most likely has an organic acidemia, which would be revealed on urinary organic acid testing.

A. Although an ammonia level would be useful for further management, it would not solidify the final diagnosis. Organic acidemias can either present with normal or elevated ammonia levels. In evaluating an infant for inborn errors of metabolism, a key point to remember is that urea cycle defects, as well as aminoacidopathies, are expected to present *without* acidosis. In urea cycle defects, the ammonia will be elevated but normal in the aminoacidopathies.

B. Although the nonspecific signs of this child may be associated with sepsis, there is no underlying fever to suggest an infectious process.

D. Congenital adrenal hyperplasia (CAH) could present with a similar clinical picture, but laboratory evaluation should reveal hyponatremia, hyperkalemia, and possibly hypoglycemia. The elevated 17-OH-progesterone level would be expected in the most common form of CAH with a 21-hydroxylase deficiency.

E. Patients with congenital hypothyroidism would not be expected to be severely acidotic unless dehydrated—a presentation of weak cry, poor feeding, and constipation would be more suggestive.

105. C. The physical exam and radiograph findings are consistent with a right-sided pneumothorax. After stabilization of the patient with attention to the ABCs (airway, breathing, circulation), a chest tube should be placed to evacuate pleural air. Barotrauma from mechanical ventilation is a risk factor for the development of a pneumothorax and is not uncommonly seen.

A. Although pneumonia may predispose a patient to a pneumothorax, there is no evidence to suggest it in this patient.

B. A confirmatory left lateral decubitus radiograph is useful in determining the extent of free air seen over the liver in an abdominal process and will also aid in detecting a more subtle pneumothorax. However, the patient is in obvious respiratory distress and has a definitively diagnostic x-ray already.

D. A confirmatory ultrasound or CT has no role in this situation.

E. The use of albuterol in this scenario is not indicated.

106. A. Extra-intestinal manifestations, such as arthritis, anemia, and erythema nodosum, are common in both forms of inflammatory bowel disease. Some of the manifestations occur only when colitis is present and some are independent of the state of the disease.

B. Colectomy is advised in patients with ulcerative colitis when there is evidence of dysplasia on surveillance biopsies that begin around 8 years after the diagnosis.

C. Fissures and fistulas are common problems in Crohn disease.

D. Continuous involvement is typically seen in ulcerative colitis; skip lesions are commonly seen in Crohn disease.

E. Upper GI involvement is not uncommon in Crohn disease and affects perhaps 30%.

107. **A.** The cause of the patient's seizures is hyponatremia. The serum sodium should be raised acutely to a level that will abort the seizure activity, typically in the range of 120 to 125 mEq/L, without being overly aggressive, which might increase the small but legitimate concern of central pontine myelinolysis caused by correcting serum sodium too rapidly. Full correction of the serum sodium acutely is therefore unnecessary. Acutely raising the sodium to 120 to 125 mEq/L in order to abort the neurologic emergency of ongoing seizure activity takes precedence over the small hypothetical risk of central pontine myelinolysis.

B. Diuretics will not affect the serum sodium acutely enough to abort ongoing seizure activity.

C. Fluid restriction would be useful in the case of syndrome of inappropriate ADH (SIADH) but has no role in this case.

D. Acutely correcting the serum sodium to 140 mEq/L increases the theoretical risk of central pontine myelinolysis as described in the explanation for A.

E. Anticonvulsants are unlikely to be helpful in the face of seizures caused by hyponatremia, which will resolve with correction of the electrolyte abnormality.

108. **B.** RSV causes inflammation of the bronchioles, which may be obstructed by edema, secretions, and cellular debris. Supportive care with oxygen, fluids, and frequent suctioning remains the mainstay of therapy for RSV.

A. Steroids have been examined in many well-controlled studies and have never shown efficacy in the treatment of RSV, unless there is underlying asthma.

C. RSV is a virus, so antibiotics will be ineffective.

D. RSV IVIG may help reduce the severity of disease if administered to at-risk populations prior to infection, but studies have not shown efficacy in the acute treatment of active RSV infection.

E. Bronchodilators have never been shown to be effective in well-controlled studies of patients with RSV, likely because the pathophysiology of the wheezing in RSV patients is caused by bronchiole plugging with secretions, edema, and cellular debris, and not from smooth muscle bronchoconstriction.

109. **A.** Blunt abdominal trauma, whether it be intentional or accidental, is a common cause of pancreatitis in the younger pediatric age group and should always be considered in the differential. Other etiologies include viral illnesses such as Epstein-Barr virus, cytomegalovirus, or coxsackie virus. Cystic fibrosis (CF) as well as a familial pancreatitis are other known etiologies.

B, C. Amylase can be normal in 10% to 15% of patients with acute pancreatitis. An elevated amylase level is not diagnostic of pancreatitis; elevated levels can be seen in salivary gland pathology such as parotitis, sialadenitis, or recurrent vomiting in eating disorders, as well as intestinal or esophageal perforation. Lipase is more specific for acute pancreatitis and typically remains elevated longer than amylase.

D. Ranson's criteria are factors that have been used to predict survival in adult patients; there are no prognostic factors developed for children. The criteria that are used at the time of admission include age greater than 55 years, leucocytosis greater than 16,000, hyperglycemia greater than 200 mg/dL, serum lactate dehydrogenase (LDH) greater than 400, and aspartate aminotransferase (AST) greater than 250.

E. Although pancreatic pseudocysts may be seen as a complication of pancreatitis, it is generally considered to be an uncommon sequela. It should be suspected in slowly improving cases of pancreatitis or when a palpable abdominal mass is detected following an acute episode.

110. | **E.** The child has stopped breathing on his own. The most important priority is to reestablish oxygenation and ventilation as suggested with 100% oxygen and bag-valve-mask.

A. Chest compressions are not necessary unless the patient is asystolic or bradycardic with a heart rate less than 60 beats per minute (BPM). The ABCs of CPR remind one to attend to airway and breathing first.

B. You have no indication of a foreign body aspiration. Abdominal thrusts are preferable to the Heimlich maneuver in children, when indicated, to avoid rib fractures.

C. A laboratory test is not necessary to tell you the patient is not breathing, and will only waste precious time before reestablishing oxygenation and ventilation.

D. You do not want to send the child anywhere out of sight for imaging in a state of extreme respiratory distress. A portable chest x-ray should be done at the bedside *after* respirations are reestablished or the patient is intubated and ventilated.

111. | **E.** This lesion may be an encephalocele, because it is in the midline and swells with crying or valsalva. Neuroimaging and neurosurgical consultation are indicated.

A. The exam findings in this newborn are descriptive of more than a simple hemangioma and deserve further investigation.

B. A biopsy would be a critical error, because the lesion could contain brain tissue.

C. The location of this lesion is suggestive that it may be much more than a hemangioma. Regardless, hemangiomas do not require steroid injection unless they are obstructing vision, the airway, or some other vital organ.

D. Massage is not helpful to either type of lesion. In addition, it is difficult to apply a pressure dressing in this location.

112. **B.** Patients with Kawasaki disease are at risk of developing coronary artery dilation and aneurysms. The goal of treatment for Kawasaki disease in the acute phase is to decrease this myocardial and coronary artery (CA) wall inflammation. The use of IVIG, in conjunction with high-dose aspirin, has been shown to decrease the progression of CA dilation and aneurysms when initiated within 10 days of the onset of symptoms.

A. Despite the initiation of treatment with IVIG and high-dose aspirin, 2% to 4% of patients will still develop CA abnormalities. ECHOs and long-term cardiology follow-up are necessary.

C. Only following the control of the acute phase is low-dose aspirin (5 mg/kg) used to prevent further CA thrombosis.

D. Steroid therapy has been shown in the past to worsen the outcome in Kawasaki disease, and is not considered standard therapy. However, in more recent literature, steroids have been reported to benefit a few patients in rare atypical cases.

E. Prolonged aspirin therapy puts the patient with Kawasaki disease at risk for Reye syndrome, especially with exposure to flu or chicken pox. Vaccines for these diseases should be given prior to hospital discharge, if not previously received.

113. **B.** The exam is most consistent with an area of cellulitis with overlying fluctuance and abscess formation.

A. Osteomyelitis to this degree would have a longer history than 5 days.

C, D. The two types of diaper dermatitis, candidal or contact, rarely cause such severe cellulitis.

E. Crohn disease does cause perirectal sinus tracts, but in this age group should present with symptoms such as diarrhea, poor weight gain, and poor growth.

114. **A.** Due to the size of this abscess, it should be incised and drained and allowed to heal secondarily. Broad-spectrum IV antibiotics that cover the common organisms (*Staphylococcus aureus, Streptococcus pyogenes*) for cellulitis, as well as those that cover anaerobes and enteric gram negatives given the location, may also be needed.

B. Simply closing up the wound with sutures would delay any further drainage.

C, D. Oral antibiotics alone or simple dressing changes with observation would not likely cure the abscess.

E. A barium enema would be painful and unnecessary in this circumstance.

115. **C.** Because the mother was adequately prophylaxed for GBS, according to American Academy of Pediatrics (AAP) guidelines the baby does not need any further work-up but should be observed for at least 48 hours. The latest guidelines further allow for possible earlier discharge at 24 hours or more if the infant is 38 weeks or older and meets all other discharge criteria with reliable follow-up.

A, B, D. Babies born at a gestational age of less than 35 weeks should have a CBC and blood culture drawn and be observed for at least 48 hours. Babies of any gestational age whose GBS-positive mothers did not receive antimicrobial prophylaxis more than 4 hours before delivery should also have a CBC and blood culture drawn and be observed for at least 48 hours. A full diagnostic septic work-up, including chest x-ray and lumbar puncture, should be guided by the physical exam and further laboratory results.

E. Empiric antibiotics should not be started before obtaining relevant cultures.

116. **C.** SOD is a rare disorder characterized by the triad of abnormal development of the optic disc, pituitary deficiencies, and often agenesis of the septum pellucidum and/or partial or complete absence of the corpus callosum. Symptoms may include blindness in one or both eyes, pupil dilation in response to light, nystagmus, seizures, hypotonia, and deficiencies of GH, adrenocorticotropic hormone (ACTH), and TSH (panhypopituitarism). Intellectual problems vary in severity among individuals. The patient described in this vignette is on glucocorticoid replacement for ACTH deficiency. As with other patients on steroid therapy, this patient needs stress dose steroids during an acute illness such as fever above 100.5°F, nausea, vomiting, etc. Stress dosing is usually two to three times the physiologic glucocorticoid dosage of 12.5 mg/m²/day.

A, E. Although patients with SOD may be on growth hormone and thyroid hormone therapies, these hormones are not adjusted during stress states and continuation of the same dosage will not have deleterious effects.

B. Patients with SOD and associated panhypopituitarism would not be expected to be on insulin therapy. Patients who require insulin therapy, most notably diabetics, may need to have insulin regimens adjusted during acute illnesses.

D. Patients with SOD may or may not have a central diabetes insipidus (DI) picture. In patients with DI, the adjustment of the vasopressin dosage during an acute illness depends upon the urine output and hydration status.

117. **C.** Respiration, heart rate, muscle tone, reflex irritability, and body color are components of the Apgar score (see Table 117). Each category is assigned a scale of 0 to 2, with scores at 1 and 5 minutes ranging from 0 to 10. The infant's Apgar score in the scenario is 4 from the following: respiration slow = 1, heart rate above 100 = 2, muscle tone limp throughout = 0, reflex irritability with grimace = 1, and pale, blue body color throughout = 0.

■ TABLE 117	Apgar Score Components		
	0	1	2
Respirations	None	Slow, irregular	Active, crying
Heart rate	None	< 100	> 100
Muscle tone	Limp	Some flexion	Active movement
Reflex irritability	None	Grimace	Crying/withdrawal
Body color	Blue	Pink body, blue extremities	Entire pink body

A, B, D, E. These are all incorrect scores. See explanation for C.

118. **C.** This child has the classic presentation of congenital adrenal hyperplasia (CAH), including ambiguous genitalia, hyperpigmentation, and salt wasting. The child is a genetic female with virilized genitalia. The most common form of CAH is 21-hydroxylase deficiency, which results in salt wasting and hyperkalemia. Low glucose is also common due to cortisol deficiency. These children often present with dehydration and even shock in the first 2 to 3 weeks of life. The treatment for CAH involves the essential replacement of cortisol and mineralocorticoids.

A. CAH is inherited as an autosomal recessive trait.

B. 21-Hydroxylase deficiency accounts for 90% of cases of CAH.

D. This child is a genetic female and does not have testes. This diagnosis should be considered in newborn infants with bilaterally nonpalpable testes.

E. Laboratory evaluation includes measurement of elevated 17-hydroxyprogesterone levels.

119. **C.** Fifteen to twenty percent of affected children have a positive family history for natal teeth. Natal teeth are seen in about 1 in 2000 newborn infants.

A. Natal teeth usually do not have a deep root system developed.

B. Natal teeth are typically located in the position of the mandibular central incisors.

D. There is a remote risk of aspiration should the tooth become dislodged. Elective extraction may be considered on an individual basis.

E. Natal teeth have been associated with other abnormalities such as cleft palate and Pierre Robin syndrome.

120. **D.** Increased intracranial pressure with a normal MRI scan and normal cerebrospinal fluid (CSF) suggests the diagnosis of pseudotumor cerebri. The treatment of pseudotumor cerebri usually involves treating the underlying condition, in this case vitamin D-deficient rickets. Breastfed babies of women who are gowned (no sun exposure) and vegetarian may develop rickets because of a lack of vitamin D in their mother's breastmilk. Pseudotumor cerebri can be due to many diseases, including those with deranged calcium and phosphorus metabolism, as well as galactosemia, hypoparathyroidism, pseudohypoparathyroidism, hypophosphatasia, prolonged corticosteroid use, excess or deficiency of vitamin A, obesity, and pregnancy. The best treatment for this baby is to provide supplements of vitamin D and calcium.

A. Some patients with increased intracranial pressure from pseudotumor cerebri are treated with serial lumbar taps to remove excessive CSF.

B, C. Acetazolamide and corticosteroids can also decrease intracranial pressure, but the underlying etiology should be treated first.

E. A neurosurgical consult would not be indicated in this case.

121. **A.** In patients with tricuspid atresia, blood is obstructed by an atretic valve and prevents flow from the right atrium to the right ventricle.

B. In tricuspid atresia, blood flows from the right atrium through a patent foramen ovale into the left atrium, then through the mitral valve to the left ventricle. In order to get to the lungs, some blood from the left ventricle passes through a VSD to the right ventricle. Shunting from the aorta to the pulmonary artery through a patent ductus is less common.

C. Because oxygenated and nonoxygenated blood mixes in the left atrium, patients with tricuspid atresia will have cyanosis in the newborn period.

D. The left ventricle has an increased load because of the right to left shunt that occurs; as a result left ventricular hypertrophy develops.

E. Treatment is aimed at improving pulmonary blood flow. Prostaglandins should be started immediately and balloon atrial septostomy may be needed as well. The goal of both palliative and definitive surgery is to assure better blood flow to the lungs.

122. **D.** Nasal CPAP may help splint the upper airway and prevent any obstructive component of apnea that may be occurring.

A. Generally, apnea of prematurity begins between the second and seventh day of life. Apnea on the first day, or beginning after the second week (or any time in a term infant), warrants immediate investigation.

B. Apnea of prematurity may respond to theophylline by mouth (PO), aminophylline (IV), or caffeine (PO).

C. Apnea associated with significant anemia may respond to packed RBC transfusion.

E. Apnea of prematurity generally resolves by 36 weeks postconceptional age (gestational age at birth plus postnatal age).

123. **D.** The dilute urine after an 8-hour overnight water deprivation is suspicious for DI. It would be dangerous to repeat a long overnight fast if this patient has DI. Therefore, a daytime water deprivation can be done lasting 7 to 8 hours with close observation for significant rise in urine concentration and serum osmolality. After 7 to 8 hours, and no significant urine concentration or rise in serum osmolality occurs, insipidus is confirmed, and the administration of vasopressin will distinguish central from nephrogenic DI. While DI is usually accompanied by hypernatremia, patients with free access to water may retain normal serum sodium concentration.

A. Vasopressin will result in urine concentration if the diagnosis is either psychogenic water drinking or central DI. Vasopressin can be used after an abnormal water deprivation test to distinguish between central and nephrogenic DI.

B. Sodium loading would be dangerous and offer no pertinent information.

C. Dilute urine after an 8-hour overnight water deprivation is suspicious for DI. It would be dangerous to repeat a long overnight fast if this patient has DI.

E. While DI is usually accompanied by hypernatremia, patients with free access to water may retain normal serum sodium concentration.

124. **A.** This is Sturge-Weber syndrome. Pulsed dye laser is frequently effective for the skin lesions and generally avoids scarring. Such therapy can begin in infancy.

B. Seizures are frequently unilateral on the contralateral side, and difficult to control.

C. For recalcitrant seizures, not well controlled with anticonvulsant medication, hemispherectomy or lobectomy has been effective, and may even prevent the development of mental retardation.

D. Glaucoma may develop with time, and therefore regular measurement of intraocular pressure is indicated.

E. Sturge-Weber syndrome is not hereditary, and is thought to result from anomalous development of the primordial vascular bed during the early stages of cerebral vascularization. The frequency of occurrence is 1 in 50,000.

125. **E.** The infant in this scenario is experiencing transient tachypnea of the newborn (TTN). TTN represents a transient pulmonary edema resulting in delayed absorption of fetal alveolar fluid secondary to a variety of risk factors that include precipitous delivery, macrosomia, and operative delivery without labor, like the infant in this scenario. Most infants recover well with only supplemental oxygen, if necessary, and observation. Obtaining a chest radiograph is a logical choice in any patient showing signs of respiratory distress. The x-ray in this scenario reveals a prominent right lobe of the thymus or sail sign that may often be confused as an infiltrate of pneumonia.

A. Although the use of oxygen will most likely not harm this patient, it is unnecessary with saturations of 98% on room air.

B. Simply administering antibiotics without obtaining cultures is generally not sound medical practice unless the patient is extremely toxic appearing.

C. Further infectious work-up should be delayed, as there are no risk factors such as prematurity, fever, or prolonged rupture of membranes. If the patient continues to not improve or worsens, then a more thorough investigation would be needed.

D. With no murmur on exam, saturations of 98% on room air, and a normal-shaped heart on x-ray, performing an ECHO at this time is not necessary.

126. **D.** The prolonged history of fever, limpness, and radiographic findings of periosteal elevation and subperiosteal fluid collection is consistent with the diagnosis of osteomyelitis. While those affected with sickle cell anemia are more susceptible to osteomyelitis with *Salmonella, Staphylococcus aureus* is still the predominant pathogen of osteomyelitis.

A. *Pseudomonas aeruginosa* infects avascular cartilaginous structures of the foot following puncture wounds.

B, C. *Salmonella* and *Brucella* tend to cause osteomyelitis of the vertebrae.

E. *Candida albicans* is not a bacterium but rather a fungus; it is an unlikely cause of osteomyelitis.

127. **C.** This patient has a hypo-osmolar serum and an inappropriately concentrated urine, diagnostic of SIADH, which may be associated with bacterial meningitis. SIADH causes the retention of free water at the level of the renal collecting tubules. The initial treatment of SIADH is to restrict administration of free water and fluid.

A. This child is probably too ill to be taking significant oral formula. However, adding additional sodium to the formula will not prevent retention of free water, and serum sodium will continue to fall.

B. Again, adding additional sodium to the IV fluids will not prevent the retention of free water caused by excess release of ADH.

D. Administration of a thiazide diuretic will result in water loss and increase sodium levels on a temporary basis, but is reserved for emergencies when sodium levels are so low that seizure activity is imminent or occurring.

E. A normal saline or hypertonic saline bolus can be helpful in patients with very severe hyponatremia (Na^+ less than 120 mEq/L) to prevent seizure activity. However, in this case fluid restriction will result in a gradual and sustained correction of the electrolytes.

128. **B.** Chest compressions in infants are correctly performed using two or three fingers placed over the lower half of the sternum coordinated in a ratio of 5:1 with respirations.

A. The heel of the hand is used in chest compressions only for a child between 1 and 8 years of age.

C. When properly performed, infant chest compressions should result in depressing the sternum to a depth of 0.5 to 1 inch.

D. The correct rate of chest compressions in an infant is *at least* 100 times per minute. The compression rate of 90 to 100 times per minute is used for children greater than 1 year of age.

E. The sternum should be compressed one third to one half of the depth of the chest in an infant, corresponding to 0.5 to 1 inch as stated in the explanation for C.

129. **D.** This child has multiple risk factors for deep venous thrombosis (DVT). They include the diagnosis of cancer, the use of asparaginase, and the presence of a central line. Venous congestion and distension are more compatible with the diagnosis of a DVT.

A. There is no erythema and/or tenderness to suggest cellulitis. Cellulitis does not typically cause venous congestion.

B. Fever and perhaps overlying erythema or fluctuance would be expected with abscess formation. Abscesses do not typically cause venous congestion as well.

C. Because this patient is reported to be in remission he should not have leukemic infiltration of his skin.

E. Fever and overlying bony tenderness should be seen with osteomyelitis of the ribs; there should be no associated venous distension.

130. | **C.** Myoglobinuria is the likely diagnosis secondary from prolonged seizure activity. The concentrated urine and normal BUN and creatinine suggest that this patient is volume depleted. It is imperative that urine flow rates be high to wash out the myoglobin and that the urine be alkaline to expedite the myoglobin excretion. Mannitol will help the urine flow while maintaining vascular volume.

A. The bolus is useful, but alkalinizing the urine and maintaining high urine volume is necessary in the treatment of rhabdomyolysis.

B. Diuresis and fluid restriction would be detrimental in myoglobinuria patients unless oliguric renal failure would ensue.

D. Diuresis and fluid restriction would be detrimental in myoglobinuria patients unless oliguric renal failure would ensue. Maintaining adequate hydration and urine flow rates may allay renal failure.

E. Although patients with rhabdomyolysis may develop acute renal failure, there is no need to begin dialysis in this patient unless the measures described in the explanation for C are unsuccessful.

131. | **C.** Addison disease occurs in about 50% of cases of adrenoleukodystrophy. When present, it generally either precedes or accompanies the onset of CNS manifestations. Occasionally Addison disease occurs without the CNS manifestations. The lab chemistries provided should be a clue to possible adrenal insufficiency.

A. Most neurodegenerative disorders are autosomal recessive. The notable exception is adrenoleukodystrophy, which is inherited as an X-linked recessive disorder.

B. The metabolic defect and/or gene mutation associated with adrenoleukodystrophy has been identified in most of the neurodegenerative disorders. In adrenoleukodystrophy there is accumulation of long-chain fatty acids due to impaired degradation in the peroxizomes due to a gene mutation on the X chromosome. In metachromatic leukodystrophy there is deficiency of arylsulfatase A activity due to a gene mutation on chromosome 22.

D. While symptomatology overlaps, adrenoleukodystrophy and metachromatic leukodystrophy are distinctly different metabolic diseases. The former results from the accumulation of very long-chain fatty acids, the latter results from the accumulation of cerebroside sulfate. Also, the former is transmitted as an X-linked trait, and the latter as an autosomal recessive trait.

E. The sphingolipidoses are caused by biochemical enzyme defects that result in the accumulation of normal lipids which cannot be sufficiently degraded.

132. **E.** Leukocyte adhesion deficiency is an autosomal recessive disorder causing recurrent bacterial infections with leukophilia without pus. In type 1 there is an absence of a surface adhesion glycoprotein on leukocytes. In type 2 there is a deficiency of a carbohydrate, which renders the neutrophils unable to adhere to endothelial cells. Delayed cord separation may occur (separation beyond 3 to 4 weeks of age).

A. Quantitative serum immunoglobulin level is a measure of B-cell function, which results in a deficiency of antibody production. Delayed umbilical cord separation is not a feature. Patients with immunoglobulin deficiencies are susceptible to infections from encapsulated organisms, such as *Streptococcus pneumoniae, Haemophilus influenzae*, and *Neisseria meningitides*.

B. Deficiencies of various complement components are generally transmitted as an autosomal trait and produce a variety of syndromes, but delayed umbilical cord separation is not a feature. Patients are more prone to invasive bacterial infections and have a higher incidence of rheumatologic disease.

C. A test of leukocyte killing is used to test for chronic granulomatous disease in which there is inability to kill catalase-positive microbes resulting in recurrent pyogenic infections and lymphadenitis. Delayed umbilical cord separation is not a feature.

D. Test for leukocyte chemotaxis is used to test for Chediak-Higashi syndrome and other syndromes associated with defective chemotaxis. These patients generally have a partial albinism, photophobia, and nystagmus; leukopenia and recurrent pyogenic infections are seen. Delayed umbilical cord separation is not a feature.

133. **E.** This patient has autosomal recessive polycystic kidney disease. Hepatic fibrosis is a common feature, and portal hypertension usually develops as patients get older. The portal hypertension and hepatomegaly may precede the renal failure. The biopsy shows diffuse cysts lined with low columnar or cuboidal epithelium representing dilated collecting ducts.

A. This is autosomal recessive polycystic kidney disease, and not sex linked.

B. Renal failure in patients with autosomal recessive polycystic kidney disease occurs at variable ages, but usually during childhood. Many have renal failure at birth or shortly thereafter.

C. Twenty-five percent of both male and female offspring will have this disorder. It is typically an autosomal recessive trait. The autosomal dominant polycystic kidney disease (adult form) will occur in 50% of offspring, both male and female.

D. The cysts of autosomal recessive polycystic kidney disease generally begin as small, dilated collecting ducts less than 2 mm in size. They may become larger as patient survival increases.

134. **F.** Cardiac defects are seen in about 60%, sterility is nearly universal in males, and mental retardation occurs in nearly all patients. This infant is exhibiting typical features of Down syndrome including hypotonia, simian creases, epicanthal folds, widely spaced first and second toes, and microcephaly. Trisomy 21, or Down syndrome, is the most common autosomal chromosomal abnormality in humans.

A. An ECHO is recommended for all patients with Down syndrome secondary to the high incidence of cardiac septal defects and endocardial cushion defects seen in these patients.

B. Sterility is seen in almost all males with Down syndrome. Some mosaic males may be fertile. Females with Down syndrome are fertile.

C. Mental retardation is common in trisomy 21 with an average IQ of 68.

D. Gastroschisis is not a common feature in Down syndrome, although intestinal atresia, especially duodenal atresia, is associated.

E. Cardiac defects are seen in about 60%, and sterility is nearly universal in males, but mental retardation occurs in nearly all patients, and is not mentioned in this option.

G. Cardiac defects are seen in about 60%, sterility is nearly universal in males, and mental retardation occurs in nearly all patients, but gastroschisis is not commonly associated with Down syndrome.

135. **D.** Diabetic ketoacidosis (DKA) is both a very serious and a very common metabolic disturbance. It can be seen in all types of diabetes mellitus, and should be considered an emergency. Its hallmark is a metabolic acidosis caused by the build-up of ketones in the blood, and it is associated with significant dehydration. Remember the ABCs and improve circulation with volume repletion before further management. The reversal of DKA requires insulin administration and rehydration. These are typically achieved with IV insulin, given as a *continuous* infusion, and with parenteral (or oral) rehydration. In addition, blood glucose levels and blood chemistries are monitored very closely throughout the course of treatment, and replacement glucose and/or electrolytes may be provided in the rehydration solution as needed.

A. DKA is treated with a continuous infusion of insulin. Using IV boluses of insulin contributes to eradicating glucose levels and will promote cerebral edema.

B. *Short-acting* insulin, given subcutaneously, can be used to reverse mild DKA on an outpatient basis, provided the patient has adequate social support, can tolerate oral rehydration, and has adequate follow-up with a physician. In contrast, *long-acting* subcutaneous insulin does *not* have a standard role in the acute reversal of DKA, given its late peak and longer duration of action.

C. Sodium bicarbonate administration has been demonstrated to be a risk factor for the development of cerebral edema in pediatric patients with DKA, and is therefore not recommended as a first-line therapy in these patients.

E. Glucagon administration would exacerbate DKA by stimulating glucose release.

136. | **D.** The infant in this scenario has clinical features consistent with transposition of the great arteries. Infants always present with cyanosis in the newborn period and a heart murmur is usually absent; a single loud S2 is often heard. Classic x-ray findings include increased pulmonary markings with an egg-shaped cardiac silhouette. Aside from attention to the ABCs with correction of an expected acidosis, prostaglandin E1 should be initiated to promote increased oxygenation by preventing ductus arteriosus closure until surgery can be performed. The lack of prenatal care in this scenario further puts the infant at risk following delivery. A prenatal ultrasound may have been beneficial in the early detection of congenital heart disease, allowing for a planned delivery at a tertiary care center.

A. Indomethacin would promote ductus arteriosus closure and would be contraindicated.

B. Captopril would be useful for afterload reduction or control of hypertension.

C. Surfactant would be indicated for premature infants with signs of respiratory distress syndrome.

E. Propranolol is a nonselective β-blocker that is used to control tachyarrhythmias and hypertension.

137. | **B.** Achalasia is a condition in which the lower esophageal sphincter fails to relax with swallowing. The cause is not clear, but pathological abnormalities of muscle fibers and ganglion cells have been seen. The average age of onset is about 10 years and many patients have problems for more than a year before properly diagnosed. Clinically, patients have vomiting, progressive difficulty swallowing, substernal pain (esophagitis), aspiration pneumonia, and growth impairment. In patients with achalasia, the barium esophagram shows a narrowed distal esophagus with proximal esophagomegaly. The diagnosis is confirmed with esophageal manometry. Treatment involves dilatation of the sphincter or surgical (Heller) myotomy. Endoscopic injection of botulinum toxin may be effective, but it is expensive and often is effective for less than 1 year. Nifedipine (calcium channel blocker) may help on a temporary basis.

A. The radiograph in hiatal hernia will show a portion of the stomach above the diaphragm.

C, D. In neither GER nor pyloric stenosis will the patient have a dilated esophagus.

E. Symptoms of esophagitis and esophageal stricture from a caustic ingestion would be of more acute onset. The slow progression of symptoms seen in this case is typical of achalasia.

138. | **C.** The AAP practice guideline for the management of acute gastroenteritis in young children states that children with diarrhea who are rehydrated should be fed age-appropriate diets.

A. Leaving a child NPO withholds needed nutrition unnecessarily.

B. The BRAT diet is too limited and is low in energy density, protein, and fat.

D, E. Similarly, clear and thick liquids will not provide adequate nutrition.

139. **C.** H-type TEFs may not be detected until later in life with recurrent pneumonias. Only 4% of TEFs are the H type. H-type TEFs have a fistula between an otherwise normal esophagus and trachea.

A. The most common type of TEF, accounting for 85% of cases, is an esophageal atresia that ends in a blind pouch with a more distal TEF. All types of TEF, other than the H type, have an associated blind esophageal pouch that accounts for the inability to pass an NG tube to the stomach.

B. There is an increased incidence of associated anomalies with TEFs, up to 50%, such as VATER/VACTERL.

D. As in the explanation for C, only 4% of TEFs are the H type.

E. Aspiration is a great risk with TEFs and prone positioning minimizes movement of gastric contents into a distal fistula.

140. **A.** Shagreen patch, subungual fibromas, and café-au-lait spots are manifestations of tuberous sclerosis. Shagreen patch is a roughened, raised, orange peel-like lesion most often seen on the thorax or lumbosacral area. Other skin lesions include adenoma sebaceum, which are angiofibromas over the nose and cheeks, which often appear between 4 and 6 years.

B. In tuberous sclerosis the degree of mental retardation is variable, and some patients, indeed, have normal intelligence. However, severe retardation and normal intelligence can occur within the same family, and the degree of retardation in the affected parent is not predictive of the offspring's intelligence. In this case, early seizures (and other early manifestations) generally are associated with more serious mental retardation.

C. Hamartomas of the kidneys and polycystic kidneys are not uncommon in tuberous sclerosis and may result in hematuria. Kidney failure may occur but is rare.

D. Phakomas of the retina are common. Phakomas are round flat gray lesions in the region of the optic disc. Mulberry tumors of the retina also occur. Cataracts would be unusual.

E. Rhabdomyomas, not myxomas, of the heart occur in about 50% of children with tuberous sclerosis.

141. **D.** Even with optimal treatment, residual abnormalities of the lower leg and foot are not unusual because there is a certain amount of deformity and atrophy to start.

A. Positional deformity of the foot is not uncommon in the newborn and is a benign condition. It must be differentiated from true clubfoot in which there is a certain amount of rigidity, atrophy, and deformity. It requires no treatment.

B. Transmission of congenital (nonsyndromic) clubfoot deformity is considered multifactorial with a major influence by a single autosomal dominant gene.

C. Treatment of clubfoot generally starts with serial casting. Surgery is generally withheld until after 3 months if adequate correction is not obtained.

E. True congenital clubfoot is characterized by some calf atrophy, and hypoplasia of the tibia, fibula, and foot bones.

142. | **D.** The findings of pneumatosis intestinalis (air in the bowel wall) and gas in the portal vein are pathognomonic for neonatal necrotizing enterocolitis (NEC). NEC is a serious medical condition that primarily affects premature infants. The intestinal mucosa becomes inflamed and necrotic and the patient develops abdominal distension, bloody stools, and bilious vomiting. They may also demonstrate lethargy, apnea and bradycardia, diarrhea, acidosis, and temperature instability. NEC can be complicated by GI tract perforation, disseminated intravascular coagulation, sepsis and shock, strictures, fistulae, and abscess formation. Treatment includes cessation of all enteral feedings, placement of an NG tube for decompression, and administration of IV fluids and broad-spectrum antibiotics. Laboratory testing should include CBC, electrolytes, clotting studies, and blood and stool cultures. Frequent abdominal radiographs are obtained to monitor improvement. Patients who fail medical management or who develop bowel perforation require surgical resection of the involved intestine.

A. In cases of suspected NEC the patient should be made NPO. Feeding intolerance following an episode of NEC is common and often necessitates the use of a protein hydrolysate formula.

B. The patient's radiograph shows evidence of NEC. It would be inappropriate to simply observe and repeat films in 24 hours.

C. As in the explanation for D, the treatment of NEC requires stopping all enteral feeds and administering IV antibiotics.

E. Although patients with NEC and free peritoneal air will require surgery, bowel resection would only be indicated in cases of bowel necrosis and/or stricture formation.

143. | **E.** About 9% of infants with Down syndrome born from mothers under 30 years old are a result of translocation, so the vast majority have trisomy 21. Of all Down syndrome babies, 95% are a result of trisomy 21, 5% a result of translocation, and 1% are mosaic.

A. While the incidence of Down syndrome in all live births is 1 in 700, there is an increased risk in subsequent pregnancies even in young mothers who have had a child with trisomy 21. It may be as high as 1%. The risk goes up to 1 in 40 in mothers over 40 years old. If the Down syndrome is caused from translocation the risk goes up to 1 in 5 live births if the mother is a balanced carrier.

B. Of all Down syndrome babies, 95% are a result of trisomy 21, 5% a result of translocation, and 1% mosaic.

C. The incidence of Down syndrome in conceptions is about twice the incidence in live births because of a high incidence of early abortions.

D. Mosaic Down syndrome results from nondisjunction in *mitosis* (cell division after meiosis). This results in two lines of cells, some with a normal chromosome complement, and some with trisomy 21. Many of these children are less severely mentally retarded.

144. | **C.** Observation only is indicated in this scenario. Healthy term infants who are exposed to varicella postnatally are not candidates for VZIG or any other treatment. They are presumed to be carrying maternal antibody, which would be protective. The 2003 Red Book would recommend VZIG be used if the infant were less than or equal to 28 weeks. (American Academy of Pediatrics. Varicella-zoster infections. In: Pickering LK, ed. Red Book: 2003 Report of the Committee on Infectious Diseases. 26th ed. Elk Grove Village, IL: American Academy of Pediatrics, 2003:679.)

A. Acyclovir is not needed in this scenario nor is it recommended in the routine treatment of chicken pox in an immunocompetent child less than 12 years of age.

B. VZIG is not recommended in this scenario. If the mother developed chicken pox 5 days before delivery up until 2 days after delivery, the infant would be a candidate for VZIG.

D. Cephazolin can sometimes be used to treat the superinfection seen with varicella skin lesions but has no role in this scenario.

E. As in the explanations for A and B, neither acyclovir nor VZIG is indicated.

145. | **E.** In patients with CF and meconium ileus, hypertonic enema solutions may be used in an attempt to relieve the intestinal obstruction; if unsuccessful, then surgical intervention is necessary.

A. Down syndrome can be associated with neonatal intestinal obstruction, specifically duodenal atresia. The radiographs will typically show a "double-bubble" sign and an absence of gas in the distal bowel. This is a very different appearance than is seen with meconium ileus. With meconium ileus, a contrast enema will demonstrate the sigmoid and ascending colon to have a small diameter and the small intestine will have air-filled dilated loops of bowel. The "ground glass" appearance on abdominal radiographs is typical.

B. Approximately 10% to 20% of children with CF will develop meconium ileus. Children with meconium ileus should always be presumed to have CF until diagnostic sweat testing or genetic testing is complete.

C. A genetic predisposition for meconium ileus has been shown. Children whose siblings had meconium ileus are more likely to develop the same condition.

D. Rupture of the bowel wall and peritonitis are known complications of meconium ileus.

146. **B.** A child in renal failure is at risk for hyperkalemia, which may cause an acute life-threatening wide-complex arrhythmia. The progressive ECG findings seen in hyperkalemia include peaked T waves, loss of the T wave, widened QRS complexes, ST segment depression, bradycardia, and ultimately ventricular dysrhythmias or asystole leading to cardiac arrest. The acute administration of calcium, either as calcium chloride or calcium gluconate, helps to protect the heart from the arrhythmogenic effect of hyperkalemia. Other helpful acute treatments include the administration of sodium bicarbonate, insulin, and glucose, and an albuterol treatment. Potassium removal can be effected either by dialysis or initially with the administration of kayexelate.

A. Anti-arrhythmic agents such as lidocaine are not very effective in suppressing the arrhythmia caused by hyperkalemia.

C, D, E. Magnesium, furosemide, and mannitol are not effective in treating this acute life-threatening arrhythmia.

147. **C.** An asthmatic patient with severe wheezing generally will respond to his oxygen need with significant hyperventilation reducing his pCO_2, and maintaining a reasonably normal pH. Here the pCO_2 is normal, and even though his pH is near normal, this would indicate he could have impending respiratory failure and should go to intensive care. Additionally, his HCO_3 is a bit on the high side, suggesting that there has been some chronic CO_2 retention.

A. The pCO_2 is below normal, suggesting he does not have impending respiratory failure. The pH is a little low, and the HCO_3 is a little low, suggesting some metabolic compensation to the hypocapnea.

B. The pCO_2 is below normal, suggesting he does not have impending respiratory failure. The pH is normal, and the HCO_3 is a little low, suggesting complete metabolic compensation to the hypocapnea.

D. The pCO_2 is below normal, suggesting he does not have impending respiratory failure. The pH is low, and the HCO_3 is also low. There is probably some metabolic compensation, but there may also be some metabolic acidosis.

E. The pCO_2 is below normal, suggesting he does not have impending respiratory failure. However, the pH is low, as is the HCO_3. While there does not seem to be respiratory failure, there is a significant superimposed metabolic acidosis.

148. **A.** Reposition the child with knees to chest. Tet spells are caused by a decrease in flow through the atretic pulmonary artery, often with exercise, crying, or feeding. This causes a relative increase in the right-to-left shunting through the VSD and worsening hypoxemia with resulting cyanosis. Holding the child in a knee-to-chest position increases systemic vascular resistance, reducing the right-to-left shunt and improving oxygenation. Ideally, the parents would be able to hold the child in this position while calming and comforting him. A second appropriate management option would include a dose of morphine to relax the child and decrease respiratory drive.

B. Oxygen would be somewhat helpful to optimize oxygenation after the right-to-left shunt is minimized, but is unlikely to be as immediately useful as the increase in systemic vascular resistance with the knee-to-chest positioning. Oxygen is, however, almost always a good idea.

C. Increased fluid volume would not address the basic problem of right-to-left shunting in the heart, and starting an IV in this child would likely increase the agitation and worsen the hypoxemia.

D. CPR is not your first choice of therapy, although a severe untreated Tet spell is life threatening.

E. The use of furosemide would be beneficial if there were signs of congestive heart failure with fluid overload, but it has no use in the management of Tet spells.

149. **D.** Diaphragmatic hernias are congenital defects of the diaphragm that allow the abdominal contents to herniate into the thorax. Large defects present in the immediate neonatal period with respiratory distress. Smaller defects may present later with feeding problems and increasing respiratory distress. The x-ray shown has opacification of the left hemithorax with some evidence of bowel gas patterns and a mediastinal shift to the right suggesting a diaphragmatic hernia.

A. Pyloric stenosis presents later, typically at age 4 to 6 weeks, with projectile vomiting and electrolyte abnormalities consisting of a hypochloremic metabolic alkalosis; a normal chest radiograph would be expected.

B. Pneumonia with pleural effusion should cause fever and an elevated WBC count.

C. TEFs present with fever, cough, and aspiration pneumonias, typically demonstrated by infiltrates in the right upper and middle lobes.

E. Duodenal atresia should present soon after delivery with bilious emesis. A classic double-bubble sign is often seen on an abdominal radiograph.

150. **A.** Diaphragmatic hernias need urgent decompression and surgical correction.

B. There is no obvious infection in this case; the use of IV antibiotics is not indicated.

C. Because there is no evidence of pneumothorax or pleural effusion, inserting a chest tube is inappropriate and would cause further problems and possible bowel perforation.

D. Pyloromyotomy is the curative surgery for pyloric stenosis.

E. An ECHO would be neither diagnostic nor therapeutic.

Setting 4: Emergency Department

Generally, patients encountered here are seeking urgent care; most are not known to you. A full range of social services is available, including rape crisis intervention, family support, child protective services, domestic violence support, psychiatric services, and security assistance backed up by local police. Complete laboratory and radiology services are available.

151. A 7-year-old boy involved in a motor vehicle accident is transported by EMS to the ER. He has been intubated because of a Glasgow coma score (GCS) of 5 at the scene and remains unconscious in the PICU, though he moves occasionally with stimulation such as suctioning. The nurse asks whether the c-collar can be removed because the c-spine films have been cleared. You answer:

A. The patient can be removed from c-spine precautions if the films have been cleared by an attending staff radiologist
B. The patient can remain in c-spine precautions by elevating the head of the bed but the collar can be removed
C. The c-spine collar can be replaced by a soft collar
D. Further studies of the c-spine (CT or MRI) would be warranted before the c-spine collar can be removed
E. A repeat set of cervical spine films will need to be obtained first

152. When a 3-year-old presented for examination, his mother expressed concern about recent clumsiness and crossing of the eyes. Of note, he has recently been suffering from headaches and a change in his gait. The pupils were noted to be equally reactive to light, and his tracking of objects was noted to be of equal quality in each eye. Of note, the amount of crossing appeared to be less with near objects than far. Which of the following would be considered the most appropriate next step in the management of this patient?

A. Head MRI with gadolinium enhancement
B. Lumbar puncture (LP) with opening pressure assessment
C. Patching of the right eye
D. Observation alone with close follow-up
E. Tensilon testing

The following 2 questions (items 153-154) relate to the same clinical scenario.

A 10-year-old boy presents to the ED with severe headache and neck pain. He has just returned from summer camp. On exam, his temperature is 38.5°C. He resists fundoscopic exam because he says the bright light makes his headache worse. He prefers to lie still and does not want to move his neck very much. There has been no trauma. A head CT was obtained and is reported as normal.

153. The most appropriate next test for diagnosis would be:

A. Serum drug screen
B. Routine urinalysis
C. MRI of the brain
D. LP
E. EEG

154. CSF exam reveals mild increase in WBCs with a predominance of lymphocytes. The glucose and protein levels in the CSF are normal. The Gram stain of the CSF shows no organisms. The most likely diagnosis is:

A. Multiple sclerosis (MS)
B. *Neisseria meningitidis* meningitis
C. Brain tumor
D. Migraine headaches
E. Aseptic meningitis

End of set

---

155. You arrive at a referring hospital to assist the transport of a 6-month-old with profuse watery diarrhea. The child has an HR of 200 BPM, sunken eyes, capillary refill of 5 seconds, appears gray, and has weak central pulses and absent peripheral pulses. The referring ED has tried over 12 times to get an IV started and has been unsuccessful. The most appropriate next step is:

A. Ask for a cutdown tray to isolate the distal saphenous vein in order to provide 20 mL/kg normal saline (NS) IV ASAP
B. Place an umbilical venous line and give 20 mL/kg IV ASAP
C. Intubate and give 20 mL/kg NS down the endotracheal tube (ETT)
D. Place a subclavian central venous line to give 20 mL/kg NS ASAP
E. Place an intraosseous line and administer 20 mL/kg NS ASAP into the bone marrow cavity

156. A 6-month-old infant presents with poor feeding, fussiness, and a heart rate of 270 to 290 BPM. She is mottled, with cool extremities and capillary refill of 5 seconds. A peripheral IV is in place in the patient's antecubital space, and all medications you might wish to administer are readily available. Which of the following interventions would be the most appropriate in the treatment of this child?

A. Administration of furosemide (Lasix) 1 mg/kg rapid IV push
B. Administration of lidocaine 1 mg/kg rapid IV push
C. Administration of warm water in a plastic bag placed suddenly over the face for 15 to 20 seconds
D. Digitalizing slowly over the next 24 hours
E. Sedation and administration of synchronized cardioversion with 0.5 J/kg

157. A previously healthy, 8-week-old female infant presents with a hypoglycemic seizure and blood sugar of 14 mg/dL. On exam she is at 95% for both weight and height, well hydrated, and healthy appearing. She has been breastfeeding every 3 hours and her mother reports a normal pregnancy with good prenatal care. Aside from the hypoglycemia, a comprehensive metabolic panel is normal. Her urinalysis showed negative ketones with no reducing substances. What is the most likely diagnosis?

A. Pneumonia
B. Adrenal insufficiency
C. Glycogen storage disease
D. Galactosemia
E. Congenital hyperinsulinism (nesidioblastosis)

158. A 4-month-old infant is brought to the ED because of constipation. The mother went back to work last week and the baby was switched from breastmilk to cow's milk formula. The parents note that for the past 2 days the baby has had some difficulty sucking his bottle. On physical exam you note that the baby has no fever but is hypotonic, has a weak cry, and seems to have an expressionless face. The baby appears well hydrated and the anterior fontanelle appears normal. How would you manage this infant?

A. Switch to a soy-based formula
B. Give 4 ounces of prune juice daily for constipation
C. Obtain consultation from a speech therapist to evaluate the sucking problem
D. Obtain laboratory tests and admit the baby to the hospital
E. Observe at home; no treatment is needed

159. A 10-year-old girl comes to the ED in July because of severe right-sided ear pain that has been getting progressively worse over the last 2 days. She has had no upper respiratory symptoms or fever. When you pull on her pinna she screams out in pain. On examination, you see a whitish discharge in the ear canal. The best treatment would be:

A. Topical antibiotic/corticosteroid otic suspension
B. IM ceftriaxone
C. Benzocaine otic solution
D. Oral amoxicillin
E. Apply warm compresses to ear

160. A 10-month-old baby comes to the ER because of a fever of 40°C. Your exam reveals that the baby has an immobile, bright red, bulging eardrum. During your exam, the baby has a generalized tonic-clonic seizure. A spinal tap shows normal CSF. You suspect that the baby had a febrile convulsion. The parents are extremely anxious and have multiple questions. Which of the following is the most accurate information to give to this boy's parents?

A. Febrile convulsions commonly occur between 9 months and 5 years of age
B. Most febrile seizures last more than 15 minutes
C. Even if there is no family history of seizures, children with simple febrile convulsions are 10 times more likely to develop epilepsy than the general population
D. Children who have a simple febrile seizure require an EEG and MRI
E. Children with two or more simple febrile seizures should routinely be given prophylactic anticonvulsant medication

161. A 5-year-old boy is seen in the ED for fever and a purpuric rash on the legs and buttocks. He has been having intermittent abdominal pain and frankly bloody stools. His right knee is warm, swollen, red, and painful. Which statement regarding this patient's condition is most accurate?

A. The cause of this condition is thought to be an IgA-mediated immune vasculitis
B. The rash tends to be on the upper extremities
C. Glomerulonephritis and arthritis are quite rare
D. The platelet count is usually depressed
E. Corticosteroids should never be used in this condition

162. A 5-year-old boy presents with a history of grossly bloody urine, puffy eyes, and headache for 1 day. His diagnostic evaluation and course were consistent with the diagnosis of poststreptococcal glomerulonephritis (PSGN). The course was benign, but 10 days after the onset his urine still contained a 3+ reaction for protein and 4+ reaction for blood on a dip stick, and a microscopic exam of his urine still revealed a full field of RBCs with many RBC casts. Which one of the following can be considered normal for uncomplicated PSGN?

    A. An elevated antistreptolysin O (ASO), which has normalized after 1 month
    B. Low serum C3 for up to 6 weeks
    C. Nephrotic syndrome within 3 months from onset
    D. Gross hematuria for up to 3 months
    E. Hypertension lasting 6 months or more

163. A 9-month-old infant is seen with a mild upper respiratory infection and is noted to have some pallor, slight icterus, and an enlarged spleen. The mother had a splenectomy for some unknown reason when she was about 6 years old. Which one of the following laboratory sets is compatible with the expected diagnosis?

    A. Hemoglobin 10.7 g/dL, MCHC 38, reticulocyte count 1.5%
    B. Hemoglobin 9.5 g/dL, MCV 80, RDW 16
    C. Total bilirubin 5.0 mg/dL, MCHC 33, RDW 13
    D. Total indirect bilirubin 0.5 mg/dL, MCHC 33, reticulocyte count 10%
    E. Hemoglobin 9.5 mg/dL, indirect bilirubin 3.5 mg/dL, RDW 10.5

164. A 2-month-old male presents to the ED with new onset seizures. The mother states that the child "rolled from the bed a couple of days ago and has not been acting right since." After discovering biparietal subdural hematomas on exam, an ophthalmic consultation is requested as the child is awaiting further head imaging. After dilating the pupils with cycloplegic eye drops, the retinas are examined. Which of the following findings would help confirm your diagnosis?

    A. White-centered, dark intraretinal hemorrhages
    B. Retinal detachment
    C. Hemorrhages scattered throughout the posterior retina only
    D. Massive bilateral eyelid ecchymoses
    E. Absence of blood within the vitreous

165. A 16-year-old female is brought into the ED by her friends. She is concerned that while at a party somebody may have put something in her drink. She is particularly concerned it may have been "the date rape drug" gamma hydroxybutyrate (GHB). Which of the following is most consistent with GHB ingestion?

    A. Hypertension, tachycardia, and diaphoresis
    B. Auditory and visual hallucinations
    C. Nystagmus, agitation, and hyperthermia
    D. Apparent coma and rapid return to consciousness when assessing a gag reflex
    E. Hyponatremia seizures after attending a rave concert

The following 2 questions (items 166-167) relate to the same clinical scenario.

A 4-year-old female presents to your pediatric ED complaining of abdominal pain for the past 3 days. The pain is diffuse, intermittent, and moderate to severe at times. Sometimes her pain is so severe that she is in tears and unable to rest comfortably; sometimes it seems to go away completely and she plays normally. Her appetite has been only slightly affected. There has not been any blood in her stools, although she has not had any stool at all for the last 3 days. Review of systems is negative for fevers, vomiting, diarrhea, sore throat, respiratory symptoms, and any other complaints. Vital signs: T, 37.0°C; HR, 96; RR, 18; BP, 100/60; pulse oximetry = 100% on room air. On exam you find a soft but full abdomen; anywhere you press, she cries. Her parents are strongly opposed to the performance of a rectal exam.

166. Which of the following is an appropriate diagnostic test to order for this patient?
   A. Order a kidneys/ureter/bladder radiograph (KUB) to assess for constipation
   B. Abdominal ultrasound to assess for appendicitis
   C. CT scan of the abdomen and pelvis to assess for appendicitis
   D. Barium enema to rule out intussusception
   E. Send home with reassurance that the abdominal pain will go away

167. The diagnostic test you selected correctly confirms your findings; what is the next step?
   A. Trial of Fleet enema to see if pain resolves
   B. Surgery consult for appendectomy
   C. Surgery consult for manual reduction of intussusception if barium enema fails to reduce it
   D. Further imaging of abdomen
   E. Outpatient GI consult in 2 months

End of set

---

168. A 4-year-old boy with a history of complex congenital heart disease presents with 4 days of fever, fatigue, anorexia, headache, and myalgias. On physical exam the boy is febrile and looks pale. He has a loud murmur and the spleen is enlarged. Laboratory tests reveal mild anemia and an elevated erythrocyte sedimentation rate (ESR). What is the most important next step in the management of this patient?
   A. Administer digoxin and furosemide
   B. Administer IV penicillin and gentamycin
   C. Administer amantadine for influenza
   D. Obtain blood cultures from multiple sites over the next 24 hours
   E. Order an ECHO

169. A 2-year-old boy with a 1-day history of abdominal pain, bloody diarrhea, and dehydration is seen in the ED. Prior to his arrival, he had a generalized seizure in the transport ambulance. On physical exam, the patient appears pale and is found to be mildly hypertensive. Several petechiae are seen on the trunk and extremities. Laboratory tests reveal anemia, thrombocytopenia, hematuria, and elevated blood urea nitrogen (BUN). The causative organism for this condition is most commonly:

A. *Staphylococcus aureus*
B. *Streptococcus pyogenes*
C. *Shigella dysenteriae*
D. Rotavirus
E. *Escherichia coli*

170. A 12-year-old with chronic liver disease presents to the ER with hematemesis of bright red blood. Her blood pressure is 74/50 with a heart rate of 120. You suspect a recurrent bleeding esophageal or gastric varice. Which of the following should be done first for the management of her upper GI bleed?

A. Send for a CBC
B. Place two IVs and give a bolus of NS (20 mL/kg)
C. Give vitamin K
D. Endotracheal intubation
E. Start an H2 blocker

171. A pediatric intern is doing a rotation in the ER when a man enters carrying a poodle. The man is complaining of crushing chest pain and then falls to the ground dropping the dog onto the lap of a 12-year-old girl waiting for her sister and mother in another room. The dog immediately yelps and bites the 12-year-old on the right ulnar aspect of the palm. The ER physician goes to the aid of the man and sends the intern to help with the 12-year-old bite victim. The 12-year-old has no past medical history and she was given diphtheria, tetanus, acellular pertussis vaccine (DTaP) when she began school. Which of the following statements is most accurate?

A. The tetanus toxoid and diphtheria toxoid (Td) are not needed
B. Prophylactic antibiotics are indicated
C. Infections caused by dog bites are almost never the result of *Pasteurella multocida*
D. Cleaning and irrigation of the wound is the most important factor in decreasing the chance of infection
E. Wounds of the hand should be sutured after thorough cleaning

172. A 13-year-old male is seen in the ED after a minor motor vehicle accident. The patient was restrained and the right-sided impact caused him to hit his head against the window without breaking it. There is no previous medical history and no family history is available as the patient is adopted. During the exam, the physician notes marked swelling of the head and neck and right side of the body. There is no bruising, erythema, itching, or hives noted. The patient is anxious and complaining of some abdominal pain. When swelling of the mouth was noted, the physician administered epinephrine without noticeable improvement. Which of the following is likely the cause for the problem?

A. Anaphylaxis to the powder in the examiner's gloves
B. Hereditary angioedema
C. Acute congestive heart failure secondary to pericardial tamponade
D. Acute septic shock secondary to bowel perforation
E. Infiltration of the IV

173. A 12-year-old female is brought to the ED by her friends after a house party. She is lethargic, confused, and has vomited. Her friends state that she simply "had too much to drink." Her lab work shows the following: Na^+, 140; K^+, 3.5; Cl^-, 95; CO_2, 18; BUN, 9; glucose, 120; measured osmolality, 350 mosm/kg; and ethanol, 120 mg/dL. What is the next step in managing this patient?

A. Call the child's parents to take her home
B. Obtain a toxic alcohol screen for methanol, ethylene glycol, and isopropyl alcohol
C. Administer IV thiamine
D. Administer IV fomepizole (4-MP)
E. Arrange for urgent hemodialysis

174. A 3-year-old child is seen in the ER with a history of fever, right-sided neck swelling, and dysphagia. His past medical history is negative and his shots are up to date. On physical exam you confirm right-sided cervical swelling with no tonsilar enlargement or uvula deviation without any evidence of stridor. He is saturating 98% on room air. A neck film is obtained (Figure 174). What would be appropriate in the management of this patient?

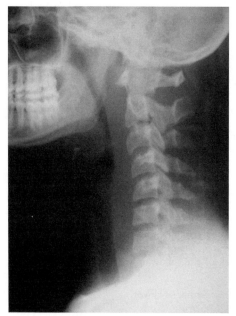

Figure 174 • Image courtesy of the Department of Radiology, Phoenix Children's Hospital, Phoenix, Arizona.

A. Immediate consultation with anesthesia and intubation in the OR
B. Administration of racemic epinephrine
C. Ear, nose, and throat (ENT) consultation for tonsillar drainage
D. Administration of ampicillin-sulbactam with ENT consult
E. Administration of dexamethasone

175. A 5-kg infant is seen in the ED with a history of profuse diarrhea. The skin has a "doughy" texture, mucous membranes are dry, extremities are cool, and capillary refill is 4 seconds. The initial serum sodium is 170 mEq/L. Which of the following is the best immediate action?

A. Infusion of D5 (0.2%) NS plus 20 mEq/L KCl at 1.5 maintenance
B. Infusion of 10 mL/kg D10W
C. Administration of 2 mEq/kg sodium bicarbonate
D. Infusion of 20 ml/kg 0.9% NaCl
E. Administration of IV antibiotics and an LP to rule out sepsis

176. A 3-year-old boy is found playing with his older brother's D-amphetamine (Adderall) tablets that he takes for ADHD. The mother has brought him to the ED for further evaluation and treatment. Which of the following clinical features would be expected should he develop toxicity?

A. Dilated pupils (mydriasis)
B. Lethargy
C. Dry skin
D. Hyponatremia
E. Constipation

177. A 25-year-old woman at 37-weeks gestation is involved in a motor vehicle accident. En route to the ED her 2.8-kg infant is delivered. Apgar scoring is 6 at 1 minute and 9 at 5 minutes. The infant is evaluated by the trauma team and no fractures are noted. The infant is admitted to the nursery. The initial evaluation of the infant by a pediatrician reveals a healthy appearing infant with a raised area on the right posterior side of the head. There is no warmth noted and very little fluctuance. The area does not appear to cross suture lines. The most likely diagnosis is:

A. Subgaleal hemorrhage
B. Normal molding given the precipitous delivery
C. Caput succedaneum
D. Cephalohematoma
E. Infection secondary to scalp monitoring in the ER

178. A 6-year-old boy is seen in the ED because of fever, sore throat, and dyspnea. You note that he is drooling and holding his neck in a hyperextended position. The boy has had no immunizations for family religious reasons. You suspect the patient has epiglottitis. Which of the following statements about epiglottitis is true?

A. The incidence of epiglottitis has decreased dramatically since the widespread use of *Haemophilus influenzae* vaccine
B. The patient should be carefully placed in the supine position, and gently restrained so that the examiner can use a tongue blade and directly inspect the epiglottis
C. Patients with epiglottitis usually have a loud barky cough
D. The classic finding on a lateral neck radiograph is called the "steeple sign"
E. Radiographs should always be performed before endotracheal intubation or tracheostomy are considered

179. A 10-year-old boy with Ewing sarcoma presents with fever and is found to be neutropenic. After a blood culture is obtained, empiric IV antibiotics are administered. Thirty minutes later, he becomes hypotensive and unresponsive. His physical exam is remarkable for bleeding gums and petechiae. His laboratory results demonstrate a low platelet count, a prolonged partial thromboplastin time (PTT) as well as prothrombin time (PT), his D-dimers are elevated, his fibrinogen is decreased, and red blood cell fragments are noted on his blood smear. The most likely diagnosis is:

    A. Disseminated intravascular coagulopathy (DIC)
    B. Immune thrombocytopenia purpura (ITP)
    C. Hemolytic uremic syndrome (HUS)
    D. Kasabach-Merritt phenomena
    E. Deep venous thrombosis (DVT)

180. A 14-year-old female presents with low-grade fever, cough, a sharp, stabbing pain over the left side of her chest extending into her left shoulder, and tachypnea. The pain is worse when she lies supine but improves with sitting upright and leaning forward. Her exam is significant for muffled heart sounds and an audible rub. A chest x-ray is obtained (Figure 180). Which of the following findings on exam/ECG would strengthen your diagnosis?

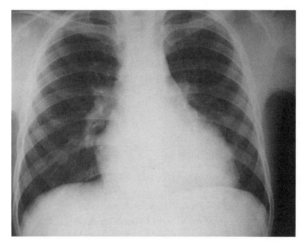

Figure 180 • Image courtesy of the Department of Radiology, Phoenix Children's Hospital, Phoenix, Arizona.

    A. Normal jugular venous distension in the neck
    B. Wide pulses
    C. Sinus bradycardia
    D. Increased pulsus paradoxus
    E. ST segment depression on the ECG
    F. Increased QRS voltage in most leads

181. A 16-year-old girl presents to the ER with complaints of "heavy" vaginal bleeding. She had menarche at the age of 13 years. Previously her menstrual cycles were regular, lasting 28 days with 5 days of bleeding. For the past 6 months, her menstrual bleeding has lasted between 7 and 11 days. She has bled through her clothes overnight. On family history, her father required multiple cauterizations for frequent epistaxis. Laboratory evaluation revealed an isolated prolongation of the PTT. Her most likely diagnosis is:

    A. Hemophilia A (factor VIII deficiency)
    B. Hemophilia B (factor IX deficiency)
    C. Lupus anticoagulant
    D. Factor XI deficiency
    E. von Willebrand disease

182. A 13-year-old presents to the ER with a history of right leg pain that is more severe at night and relieved by ibuprofen. His physical exam is essentially normal with no limp and some mild tenderness over the lower tibial region. A radiograph is obtained (Figure 182A). Which of the following is the most likely diagnosis?

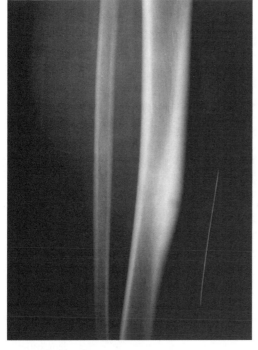

Figure 182A • Image courtesy of the Department of Radiology, Phoenix Children's Hospital, Phoenix, Arizona.

    A. Growing pains
    B. Osteomyelitis
    C. Osteosarcoma
    D. Osteoid ostoma
    E. Eosinophilic granuloma

183. A 14-year-old male has been brought into the ER following a syncopal episode. He was getting up from the toilet and reported feeling dizzy and then blacking out. His past medical and family history are unremarkable. His physical exam is completely normal as is an ECG strip obtained during his ambulance ride over. Which of the following would be an appropriate work-up at this point?

A. Discharge home and follow-up with cardiology for a 24-hour Holter monitor
B. Admission to the ICU for inpatient monitoring
C. STAT ECHO in the ED
D. Placement of arterial line in the ED
E. Psychiatry or psychology referral

184. A 2-year-old child is brought into the ER by his mother. She reports that he was found in the bathroom with his grandmother's "iron pills" all around the floor. The mother is frantic, and to reassure her you counsel her that which of the following, once confirmed, virtually excludes the diagnosis of iron poisoning?

A. The absence of emesis 6 hours postingestion
B. Normal basic metabolic profile 1 hour postingestion
C. An alert playful, age-appropriate child
D. The absence of leukocytosis 1 hour postingestion
E. The lack of radiolucent material on an abdominal x-ray

185. An 8-year-old male was an unrestrained front-seat passenger in an automobile accident. He was found by the paramedics in front of the car bleeding from the scalp, nose, and left lower leg. He presents with nasal flaring, intercostal retractions, and tachypnea. His pupils are reactive to light, he opens his eyes to pain, and groans with painful stimuli. His vital signs are temperature 36°C, pulse in the field 200, which has decreased to 170 with fluid, respiratory rate 60, and blood pressure 80/40. His extremities are cool, with thready pulses and capillary refill of 5 seconds. He has already received two 20 mL/kg NS infusions. He is in c-spine precautions. Which of the following interventions is most appropriate to perform first at this time?

A. Directly admit the patient to the PICU for close observation
B. Obtain an abdominal CT
C. Order a CT scan of the head
D. Repeat 20 mL/kg 0.9% NS IV
E. Placement of a femoral central venous line for central venous pressure assessment of intravascular fluid volume

186. A 4-year-old boy presents to the ED with a history of right lower quadrant abdominal pain that has been present for about 24 hours. The onset of the pain was followed by development of low-grade fever and vomiting. The patient has had no diarrhea but is not eating at all. Over the past 3 to 4 hours, the patient's pain has become more generalized and the abdomen has become distended. On physical exam the patient demonstrates generalized rebound tenderness, absent bowel sounds, and moderate dehydration. The best next step in the management of this patient is:

A. Take the patient to the OR for immediate appendectomy
B. Admit to the hospital and start oral rehydration solution
C. Start IV fluids; no antibiotics necessary
D. Start IV fluids and broad-spectrum antibiotics
E. Obtain stool specimen for microscopic examination and culture

187. A previously healthy, term 15-month-old male presents to the ER with a history of the sudden onset of rectal bleeding. The parents deny fever, vomiting, diarrhea, or abdominal pain. He has had three episodes of bright red blood per rectum. Hemodynamically, he is stable and his initial hemoglobin is 11. Which of the following tests is most likely to give you the correct diagnosis?

A. Flat plate x-ray (KUB) of the abdomen
B. Abdominal ultrasound
C. Meckel scan
D. CT of the abdomen
E. Upper GI

188. A 3-year-old girl comes to the ED because of fever, ear pain, protruding pinna, and erythematous, tender swelling in the postauricular area. There is also evidence of acute otitis media with a red, immobile, bulging tympanic membrane (TM). The patient has no signs or symptoms of meningitis. The best initial management option is:

A. Oral amoxicillin for 10 to 14 days
B. IM ceftriaxone for 3 consecutive days as an outpatient
C. Hospitalize for IV cefuroxime
D. Hospitalize for IV ampicillin-sulbactam and myringotomy
E. Arrange for otolaryngologist to perform mastoidectomy

189. A 10-month-old child is found playing with his mother's medicine bottles. There are some tablets on his shirt and some white powder around his mouth. His parents decide to take him to the ED. On arrival in the ED, the child is clearly symptomatic with a dry mouth, agitation, tachycardia, flushed skin, and hyperthermia. You would be most suspicious of which of the following medications:

A. Acetaminophen
B. Propranolol
C. Diphenhydramine (Benadryl)
D. Lithium
E. Phenytoin

190. A 16-year-old female is brought to the ER by her parents. They report that she went out with friends earlier and now has a high fever and is quite jumpy. The ER doctor examines the patient and finds her to be agitated with a heart rate of 122 and a temperature of 101°F. Her pupils are dilated, and she is diaphoretic. The patient has an infant's pacifier tied around her neck. While examining the patient, two pills with a cartoon character stamp fall out of her shirt pocket. The physician asks the parents if there has ever been a problem with illegal drug use, specifically MDMA or "ecstasy." Which of the following would be an appropriate next step for the physician?

A. Await lab analysis of the two unidentified pills
B. Administer syrup of ipecac
C. Obtain IV, and monitor airway and circulation
D. Allow patient to "detox" in the ER
E. Have emergency team locate friends for pill identification

191. A mother brings her 7-month-old baby to the ER because he has been pulling at his right ear for the last 2 to 3 weeks. The child is otherwise healthy with no symptoms of upper respiratory infection (URI), vomiting, diarrhea, or fever. On physical exam, the right TM is moderately erythematous, but no bulging or retraction is noted. Pneumatic otoscopy reveals normal mobility. The most likely diagnosis is:

A. Early acute otitis media
B. Otitis media with effusion (OME)
C. Bullous myringitis
D. Normal ears
E. Perforated TM

The following 2 questions (items 192-193) relate to the same clinical scenario.

You are evaluating an 8-year-old boy in the ED for a painful right great toe. He stubbed it playing soccer 15 days ago. Since then, he has had increasing pain, redness, and swelling of this toe. On exam, he is febrile to 38.9°C and cannot walk because of the pain in his toe. The toe is purplish-red, swollen, and the nail bed is broken.

192. The most appropriate next step in management would be:

A. MRI of the right foot
B. Whole-body bone scan
C. CBC, blood culture, and plain films of the right foot
D. Splint application and discharge for outpatient follow-up
E. IV oxacillin

193. After review of the lab and x-ray results, you note that his white count is elevated with a majority of neutrophils and that the radiologist's dictation mentions "significant soft tissue swelling with a subperiosteal fluid collection around the base of the distal phalanx of the right great toe." The most likely diagnosis is:

A. Osteomyelitis of the right great toe
B. Cellulitis of the right foot
C. Avulsion of the right great toe nail bed
D. Right ankle sprain
E. Acute lymphoblastic leukemia (ALL)

End of set

---

194. A 9-year-old girl with a known seizure disorder is brought to the ED for evaluation of prolonged hemiparesis following one of her typical focal left-sided seizures. She had been at summer camp and had neglected to take her routine medicine for seizure control. On exam, she is appropriate but drowsy. Her neurologic exam is significant for left-sided weakness and a positive Babinski reflex on the left. You suspect a diagnosis of Todd paralysis. The most appropriate next step in management is:

A. Cerebral angiogram
B. Admission to the PICU with neurosurgical consultation
C. Head MRI/MRA
D. Admission to the pediatric ward for 24-hour observation
E. LP

195. A 2-year-old girl is brought to the ED for difficulty breathing. She had been well earlier in the day. The mother states that the child had a coughing fit after she came out of her brother's room. When the mother investigated, she found the brother's piggy bank broken open on the floor. The girl has no significant past medical history. On exam, she is tachypneic and has wheezes over her right hemithorax. You suspect a foreign body aspiration. The most appropriate imaging study to confirm the diagnosis would be:

A. Contrast-enhanced CT of the chest
B. Plain films of the chest and neck
C. Modified barium swallow with speech pathology present
D. Upper GI series
E. Cervical spine x-rays

196. A 6-month-old infant is brought into the ED following a fall to a wooden floor from his mother's bed, which occurred 20 minutes ago. The child did not lose consciousness from the event and has been behaving appropriately. On physical exam you notice a mild swelling over the left parietal region as well as significant head lag with poor truncal tone. A skull radiograph has been previously ordered by the resident and is available for your review (Figure 196). Your next step in the management of this patient should include:

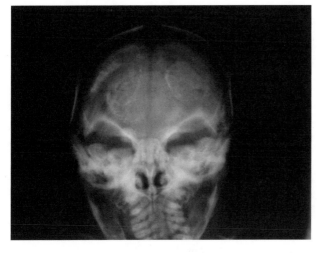

Figure 196 • Image courtesy of the Department of Radiology, Phoenix Children's Hospital, Phoenix, Arizona.

A. Immediate neurosurgical consultation
B. MRI of the head
C. Discharge to the custody of child protective services
D. Admit to the hospital for overnight observation
E. Admit to the hospital for a more detailed evaluation

197. A 15-year-old male presents to the ED with a history of agitation and tachycardia. His friends say he is "on something" but refuse to say anything more. Myocardial ischemia secondary to this drug may be worsened with a β-blocker:

   A. Cocaine
   B. Amphetamine
   C. PCP
   D. Heroin
   E. Codeine

The following 3 questions (items 198-200) relate to the same clinical scenario.

A 2-month-old girl is brought to the ED for evaluation after she fell out of her car seat off a table and landed on a concrete floor. She cried immediately, but over the next 4 hours got progressively drowsy and was not interested in feeding. On exam her vital signs are all within normal limits; however, she does have a 2-cm oval raised hematoma over her left parietal bone. The rest of the exam is normal.

198. The best next step in management would be:

   A. Skull radiography
   B. Head CT
   C. Head MRI
   D. Bone scan
   E. Head ultrasound

199. The appropriate imaging study reviewed by yourself and the housestaff reveals a linear, nondepressed skull fracture. The best next step in management would be:

   A. Discharge to a teenage relative while the parents are at work
   B. Discharge to the parents who can observe the baby at home
   C. Admission to the hospital for 24-hour observation
   D. Neurosurgical consultation
   E. Rapid sequence intubation and hyperventilation

200. You are beginning to write up the appropriate paperwork for your patient when the radiologist calls with his interpretation of the study: "A depressed skull fracture of 6-mm depth over the left parietal bone with no obvious intracranial injury." Following this information, the best next step in management would be:

   A. Discharge to a teenage relative while the parents are at work
   B. Discharge to the parents who can observe the baby at home
   C. Admission to the hospital for 24-hour observation
   D. Neurosurgical consultation
   E. Rapid sequence intubation and hyperventilation

End of set

Answers and Explanations

Answer Key

151.	D	168.	D	185.	D
152.	A	169.	E	186.	D
153.	D	170.	B	187.	C
154.	E	171.	D	188.	D
155.	E	172.	B	189.	C
156.	E	173.	B	190.	C
157.	E	174.	D	191.	D
158.	D	175.	D	192.	C
159.	A	176.	A	193.	A
160.	A	177.	D	194.	D
161.	A	178.	A	195.	B
162.	B	179.	A	196.	E
163.	B	180.	D	197.	A
164.	A	181.	E	198.	B
165.	D	182.	D	199.	C
166.	A	183.	A	200.	D
167.	A	184.	A		

151. **D.** A child can have spinal cord injury without radiologic abnormality (SCI-WORA), where the spinal cord has been damaged but the cervical vertebrae appear normal by x-ray. Therefore, a pediatric patient's c-spine should only be cleared when both the c-spine radiographs are normal *and* a clinical exam of the neck and spine can be reliably performed. If such a clinical exam cannot be performed, then further evaluation of the cervical spinal cord, such as with CT or MRI, would need to be performed to rule out the possibility of SCIWORA.

A, B, C, E. See explanation for **D.**

152. **A.** Elevated intracranial pressure is quite likely in this case. Crossing of the eyes, which is worse with distant gaze than near gaze, typifies a sixth nerve palsy. Active abduction is needed to maintain the straightness of the eyes at a distance, but not at closeness. The symptoms of possible ataxia with a history of recent clumsiness are concerning for a posterior fossa mass and warrant further investigation with a head MRI.

B. Prior to sampling the cerebral spinal pressure, the possibility of herniation from the pressure drop should be eliminated by cranial imaging.

C. Patching is indicated for the treatment of amblyopia, commonly associated with strabismus. In such cases, the unaffected eye is patched to force or stimulate the use of the amblyopic eye.

D. Given the constellation of symptoms in this patient, observation alone would not be appropriate.

E. Tensilon testing for myasthenia gravis is unnecessary as it is not a likely source of this set of symptoms. Myasthenia is quite unusual in this age group, and while it often presents with strabismus, gait issues are quite unusual as well.

153. **D.** This boy presents with signs of meningitis, which include nuchal rigidity and/or pain, photophobia, and an associated fever; an LP would be the appropriate next step in management.

A, B, E. A serum drug screen, routine urinalysis, and EEG would not reveal any information about his CSF or meninges.

C. MRI of the brain, after a normal head CT scan, would be costly, delay appropriate treatment, and not provide any useful, additional information.

154. **E.** This is the typical pediatric presentation of aseptic meningitis in late summer: headache, neck pain/stiffness, photophobia, and CSF findings showing an increased WBC count with a predominance of lymphocytes with a normal CSF glucose and protein.

A. MS is a slowly progressive neurologic disease with insidious onset, not acute as in this case.

B. If *Neisseria meningitidis* were the cause of his illness, the patient would be expected to be sicker and have CSF findings more consistent with a bacterial process:

increased WBC count with a predominance of neutrophils and increased protein with a decreased glucose.

C. A brain tumor should have been seen on the head CT and would not be expected to present with fever and neck pain.

D. Migraine headaches would not be expected to produce fever and the CSF findings seen in this patient, although associated photophobia and neck pain may occasionally be seen.

155. E. The child presented is in significant shock, manifested by gray color, prolonged capillary refill, absent peripheral pulses, and weak central pulses. This child needs vascular access immediately before bradycardia and irreversible cardiac arrest occurs. If IV access cannot be readily and *immediately* obtained, a needle should be inserted into the bone marrow cavity and rapid fluid resuscitation initiated. The usual location for intraosseous access is the proximal tibia, just below the tibial tuberosity, but any bone marrow access can be utilized in such an emergency (such as the humerus, anterior or posterior ileac crest, etc.). Fluid resuscitation can be ongoing through this site while attempts at securing further vascular access via a cutdown, central line, or peripheral vein ensue.

A. A cutdown procedure to isolate the saphenous vein may be necessary if no other IV access can be obtained. However, an intraosseous (IO) line is much easier to place and allows much more rapid treatment for this gravely ill child.

B. An umbilical venous line can be used in premature infants and neonates, but would not be possible in a 6-month-old child.

C. The primary problem in this patient is circulatory shock, not respiratory compromise. With proper fluid resuscitation, intubation and ventilation may be avoided.

D. Placement of a subclavian line is not the first choice in a 6-month-old infant. Intraosseous line placement is the appropriate first step.

156. E. The scenario presented above describes a child with supraventricular tachycardia (SVT) who is *unstable* and in shock. The shock is manifested by cool extremities, mottled skin color, and prolonged capillary refill. Synchronized cardioversion is the first-line treatment of SVT in an unstable patient with hypotension.

A. Furosemide (Lasix) would be an effective treatment for a patient with evidence of congestive heart failure and fluid overload with pulmonary edema. It has no role for the initial treatment of SVT.

B. Lidocaine is a group-1B antiarrhythmic drug that is indicated for the treatment of acute ventricular arrhythmias, most commonly that of ventricular fibrillation. Adenosine is considered the drug of choice when treating SVT.

C. Administration of ice and water increases vagal tone, which will also slow conduction in the atrioventricular (AV) node and can result in rapid conversion of SVT. The use of warm water would have the opposite intended effect of tachycardia.

D. Digitalizing slowly over 24 hours is not an appropriate choice for someone who is unstable and in shock because it does not correct the dysrhythmia rapidly enough.

Once the child has been converted to a stable rhythm, digitalization can be started to reduce the risk of subsequent events.

157. **E.** This patient has a ketone-negative hypoglycemia without failure to thrive. Congenital hyperinsulinism is the most likely diagnosis. An uninterrupted flow of glucose in the blood is essential for normal brain metabolism. Categories of hypoglycemia include abnormalities in hormonal regulation, inborn errors of glucose, fat, or protein metabolism, prematurity, drugs, organ failures, and certain neoplasms. Hormonal conditions include deficiencies in the growth hormonal axis, adrenal hormonal axis, thyroid hormonal axis, or insulin hormone excess.

The algorithm below can be useful in helping to diagnose hypoglycemic disorders:

Ketotic

High lactate
→ Inborn errors of glucose metabolism

Normal lactate
→ Glycogen storage diseases, hormonal deficiency, ketotic hypoglycemia

Nonketotic

Reducing substances
→ Hereditary fructose intolerance, galactosemia

No reducing substances
→ Hyperinsulinism, fatty acid oxidation defect, drugs

A. The patient is not noted to have tachypnea, cough, or fever, and thus pneumonia is unlikely.

B. Adrenal insufficiency should present with electrolyte abnormalities, most notably hyponatremia and hyperkalemia, as well as ketonuria if hypoglycemic.

C. Patients with glycogen storage disease often present with hepatomegaly and failure to thrive, and would be expected to be able to produce ketones.

D. Galactosemia is a disorder of carbohydrate, specifically galactose metabolism. Infants often present with jaundice, failure to thrive, hepatomegaly, and hypoglycemia. Negative ketones, but positive reducing substances, would be expected on a urinalysis.

158. **D.** This is a classic case of infant botulism. Babies with this condition are listless and hypotonic and may have a weak cry, poor head control, feeding difficulties, and constipation. As in this case, there is often a recent change in feeding practice. Additionally, honey has been implicated as a cause in several cases. In adult cases of botulism, the patient swallows the toxin from improperly prepared foods, but infants become infected by ingesting *Clostridium botulinum* spores that colonize in the baby's colon. Because paralysis of the respiratory muscles can cause respiratory failure, these babies must be admitted to the hospital for careful supportive care, which may include endotracheal intubation. Antibiotics are not helpful. Stools should be tested for botulinum toxin.

A. Cow's milk allergy or intolerance generally causes diarrhea, not constipation, and would not account for difficulties in suck and hypotonia.

B. The natural sugars in prune juice can act to draw water into the gut lumen and help hydrate and soften stools. In this case of botulism, the constipation is toxin mediated and stool softeners would not be effective.

C. This baby may be too ill for a speech therapy evaluation at this time. The gag, suck, and swallowing reflexes begin to return to normal after approximately 1 to 3 weeks. At that time, the speech therapist can be helpful with decisions regarding resumption of oral feedings.

E. Infant botulism can be fatal. When the condition is recognized early and babies get adequate supportive care and proper airway management in the hospital, the mortality rate is less than 5%.

---

159. **A.** During the summer, many children who go swimming develop external otitis, also known as "swimmer's ear." This condition is due to maceration of the ear canal epithelium caused by moisture or chemical irritation. The pain can be intense, especially with manipulation of the pinna or pressure on the tragus. Unlike acute otitis media, most cases are not associated with signs or symptoms of an upper respiratory condition. Secondary bacterial infection is common with external otitis. The best treatment for most cases is a topical combination antibiotic-steroid suspension that is instilled into the ear canal for about 7 to 10 days. For prevention, the ear canals should always be dried well after swimming. Some experts also suggest acetic acid (vinegar) for prophylaxis.

B. Systemic antibiotics, such as ceftriaxone, are not necessary for external otitis.

C. Drops containing benzocaine can be effective in reducing pain, but will not help with the infection or inflammation seen in external otitis.

D. Topical treatment is adequate. Oral agents such amoxicillin can be associated with unnecessary systemic side effects, such as diarrhea or rash.

E. Because the pain originates from the ear canal, warm compresses to the external ear would not help.

---

160. **A.** It is true that most febrile seizures occur between 9 months and 5 years of age.

B. Febrile convulsions are considered "atypical" if they last longer than 15 minutes, occur multiple times in the same day, or are associated with focal seizure activity or focal neurologic findings. If a child has "atypical " seizures, a family history of epilepsy, seizure onset before 9 months, delayed development, or preexisting neurologic disease, there will be greater risk for developing epilepsy later.

C. Children with a typical simple febrile convulsion without risk factors are not significantly more likely to develop epilepsy than the general population.

D. While it is extremely important to rule out meningitis, an extensive diagnostic work-up with serum electrolytes, toxicology screening, an EEG, or neuroimaging is not recommended in children with a simple febrile seizure.

E. Prolonged anticonvulsant prophylaxis is not recommended for simple febrile seizures. Some experts feel diazepam (Valium) may be given at the onset of a febrile illness to children with a history of very frequent recurrences of simple febrile seizures.

161. **A.** The case history is a typical presentation of Henoch-Schönlein purpura (HSP). Most cases are preceded by a viral infection and the symptoms are secondary to an immune-mediated vasculitis involving IgA antibodies and complexes.

B. The rash tends to be crops of palpable purpuric lesions that have a predilection for the buttocks and lower extremities.

C. In addition to the rash, arthritis, glomerulonephritis, hypertension, and abdominal pain are common.

D. As opposed to idiopathic thrombocytopenic purpura, the platelet count in HSP is normal or elevated.

E. The abdominal pain is sometimes associated with intussusception, which should be considered whenever the abdominal pain is severe or if the stools are grossly bloody (currant jelly stools). Many patients with HSP have a mild illness and do not require hospitalization. Severe abdominal pain, renal disease, and hypertension are criteria for admission. Corticosteroids may help abdominal pain due to intestinal vasculitis. Their use may also prevent serious chronic renal disease.

162. **B.** The C3 is low early in the course of PSGN, but in all cases returns to normal in 6 to 8 weeks. A persistently low C3 suggests a different type of hypocomplementemic glomerulonephritis.

A. ASO is usually elevated early and frequently remains high for 3 to 6 months. When PSGN is secondary to skin infection the anti-DNAase B is often more strongly positive.

C. Diminishing significant proteinuria can last as long as 3 months, but heavy proteinuria with or without nephritic syndrome suggests a complicated course and warrants reevaluation.

D. While gross hematuria is a common initial finding, this should gradually disappear in 2 to 3 weeks.

E. Hypertension is common during the acute phase of PSGN, but it should not persist as the urine clears and the other symptoms abate.

163. **B.** The diagnosis is most likely hereditary spherocytosis. The findings of anemia, normal MCV, and high RDW are all compatible with the diagnosis of hereditary spherocytosis.

A. The diagnosis is most likely hereditary spherocytosis. The findings of anemia and high MCHC are compatible with the diagnosis of hereditary spherocytosis, but the absence of reticulocytosis would be unusual in a hemolytic process.

C. The diagnosis is most likely hereditary spherocytosis. The anemia is hemolytic, and the finding of both a high MCHC (above 35) and a high RDW (over 14.5) is almost pathognomonic of this disease. Anemia, reticulocytosis, and an elevated indirect bilirubin are the rule. Therefore this selection, which includes a normal MCHC and RDW, is not compatible with the diagnosis of hereditary spherocytosis.

D. A normal direct bilirubin and high reticulocyte count both occur in hereditary spherocytosis. However, you would expect the *indirect* bilirubin to be elevated. The normal MCHC is also expected and is not of any clinical assistance in making the diagnosis.

E. The diagnosis is most likely hereditary spherocytosis. The findings of anemia and high indirect bilirubin both support the diagnosis of hemolytic anemia. However, the RDW should be high in hemolytic anemia.

164. | **A.** The delay in treatment and suspicious story of a 2-month-old being unattended and rolling off a bed are highly suggestive of abuse. The infant in this scenario should have a thorough physical exam for abuse as well as diagnostic studies to include a head CT, skeletal survey, and retinal exam. Shaken baby syndrome, which manifests as subdural hematomas and retinal hemorrhages, is a concern in this case. After several days, the yellow centers of intraretinal hemorrhages, so typical of shaken baby syndrome, begin to turn white or gray.

B. Retinoschisis, a splitting of the layers of the retina, rather than detachment, is only rarely seen spontaneously.

C. Shaken baby syndrome is typified by hemorrhages of multiple layers of the retina, and multiple areas from posterior to anterior.

D. Shaken baby syndrome is typified by a normal examination of the external eye, and internal eye hemorrhaging.

E. Bridging retinal vessels and subarachnoid sources can produce marked vitreal bleeding in shaken baby syndrome.

165. | **D.** GHB is a concern for potential abuse as a date rape drug. Although the mechanism of action of GHB is not clearly understood, GHB appears to influence dopaminergic activity, probably by GHB receptors. A clue to the diagnosis of GHB is an apparent coma with a rapid return to consciousness when stimulated (usually when attempting to intubate).

A. Hypertension, tachycardia, and diaphoresis may be seen following the ingestion of sympathemetic drugs such as cocaine or methamphetamine.

B. Auditory and visual hallucinations would be more consistent with phencyclidine (PCP).

C. Nystagmus, agitation, and hyperthermia may be seen following excessive diphenhydramine (Benadryl) ingestion.

E. Ecstasy ingestion would be more typical with a presentation of hyponatremic seizures after a rave concert, most likely secondary to the excessive drinking of water in an effort to stay hydrated from prolonged dancing.

166. **A.** The patient's clinical presentation is consistent with constipation-induced abdominal pain, which is a common mimic for appendicitis in the pediatric age range. Factors suggesting against appendicitis in this case are:
- No fevers despite 4 days of symptoms
- Intermittent pain that sometimes is severe, and at other times goes away completely
- No significant change in appetite
- No vomiting

If a rectal exam had been performed that confirmed the presence of a large amount of stool in the vault, a KUB would not be necessary before a therapeutic trial of an enema. However, in this case, it is quite justifiable to obtain a KUB to confirm the presence of increased fecal material.

B, C. The above-listed factors argue against appendicitis and the need for a CT scan or an ultrasound.

D. Intussusception would certainly be high in the differential if this patient were between 6 months and 2 years of age. Although it can occur in older children, it is much less common. In this patient with no blood in her stools, it would be more reasonable to exclude constipation first before embarking upon a more extensive work-up.

E. Simple reassurance would not be appropriate in this patient.

167. **A.** Typically, when a Fleet enema is given and a large stool results, the patient who was previously writhing in pain now becomes quite happy and comfortable and no further work-up or consultation is needed. However, if such a patient stools after an enema but still has significant abdominal pain, further work-up is necessary, as the presence of constipation does not rule out more serious etiologies of abdominal pain.

B, C. A surgical consult would not be necessary in this patient with constipation.

D. Further imaging of the abdomen would most likely not be necessary unless severe pain persists as described in the explanation for A.

E. Although patients with a chronic history of constipation may need further GI involvement, it would be inappropriate to refer a patient to subspecialty care without initial interventions of dietary change and the use of stool softeners and/or laxatives. It is unlikely that the patient in this scenario, who has no significant past medical history, will need subspecialty involvement in the near future.

168. **D.** A presumptive diagnosis of infective endocarditis is made whenever a patient with underlying heart disease has an unexplained fever for several days' duration associated with typical clinical findings. Patients may have a new murmur or an increased intensity of an existing murmur. There may be petechiae of the skin, mucous membranes, or conjunctiva, but the classic Osler nodes, Janeway lesions, and splinter hemorrhages are rare. Embolic complications include pulmonary emboli, hematuria and renal failure, and seizures or hemiparesis. Patients generally require treatment with at least 4 to 6 weeks of IV antibiotics. *Streptococcus viridans, Staphylococcus aureus*, and group D streptococcus (enterococcus) are responsible for 90% of cases of infectious endocarditis. The diagnosis is generally made by isolation of these organisms from blood culture. The timing of the blood cultures is not important because the bacteremia is constant.

A. This patient is not in cardiac failure and does not require digoxin or furosemide.

B. Antibiotic pretreatment significantly decreases the chance of isolating the organism, so antibiotics should not be given prior to obtaining cultures.

C. While some of the symptoms are similar to those seen in influenza, this patient's history, physical exam, and lab results are more typical of infectious endocarditis. Amantadine would not be beneficial.

E. An ECHO may show the vegetation, but a normal ECHO does not rule out the possibility of endocarditis. Small vegetations early in the course of the disease may not be detected.

169. **E.** This patient's clinical presentation is typical of hemolytic-uremic syndrome (HUS). Many cases follow ingestion of poorly cooked hamburger meat that contains a toxin produced by *E. coli* O157:H7. The syndrome consists of microangopathic hemolytic anemia, thrombocytopenia, and acute renal failure. Patients may develop toxic megacolon, bowel wall necrosis, intussusception, and/or bowel perforation. Many patients have CNS findings such as irritability, lethargy, coma, seizures, or hallucinations. Thrombotic or hemorrhagic stroke may occur. Chronic renal insufficiency occurs in 5% to 10% of patients. The blood smear in HUS shows fragmented red blood cells or schistocytes. Historically, 10% to 20% of patients with *E. coli* O157:H7 infection develop HUS. Recently, it has been shown that administration of antibiotics to patients with *E. coli* infection can actually increase the chance of developing HUS. Treatment includes supportive care to manage fluid and electrolyte imbalance, hypertension, anemia, and bleeding. Renal dialysis is necessary in 30% to 50% of patients.

A. *Staphylococcus aureus* can produce a clinical picture consistent with food poisoning, but is typically not associated with HUS. *S. aureus* is further associated as a causative organism in toxic shock syndrome, scalded skin syndrome, pneumonia, osteomyelitis, arthritis, cellulitis, and other localized skin infections.

B. *Streptococcus pyogenes* is responsible for causing cellulitis and other localized skin infections, as well as arthritis, osteomyelitis, and, less commonly, toxic shock syndrome.

C. *Shigella dysenteriae* infection can result in HUS, but less commonly than *E. coli*. Patients with *S. dysenteriae* typically present with bloody diarrhea and systemic symptoms of fever, vomiting, and abdominal pain. Treatment with a third-generation cephalosporin is recommended and shortens the duration of illness.

D. Rotavirus is a common cause of diarrhea in the pediatric population and often produces diffuse, foul-smelling, water loss stools. It does not commonly cause bloody diarrhea and/or HUS.

170. | **B.** In any unstable patient with an upper GI bleed, the first step is to place two IVs and give volume resuscitation.

A. Following the establishment of IV access, attempts are made to type and screen/cross blood for transfusion and perform further diagnostic testing.

C. Vitamin K may be helpful in patients with a known elevated prothrombin time (PT) but the effect is not immediate.

D. Endotracheal intubation is needed infrequently only in those patients who develop altered level of consciousness due to rapid blood loss.

E. The use of an H2 blocker while the patient remains with nothing by mouth (NPO) or for the treatment of suspected ulcer may be useful, but it is not the first step in management of the patient with an upper GI bleed.

171. | **D.** Irrigation and cleaning is the mainstay of wound management.

A. In this case Td is indicated given that more than 5 years have passed since vaccination.

B. Prophylactic antibiotics are not necessary. The wound should be monitored for further signs of infection and antibiotics prescribed if then necessary.

C. Early infections are often caused by *Pasteurella multocida* in both cat and dog bites.

E. Suturing of the hand, particularly following a dog bite, should be avoided if at all possible given the higher chance of infection.

172. | **B.** Hereditary angioedema is an autosomal dominant defect in the complement system. Angioedema that does not respond to epinephrine and is not associated with hives should be the clue to the health care provider. Often there is a family history of edema associated with minor trauma and/or stress. The differential would include anaphylaxis, but one should see some resolution with epinephrine in that case.

A. Anaphylaxis to the gloves' powder would be expected to be more generalized and should respond to epinephrine.

C. There is no history of blunt chest trauma or signs on physical exam, such as muffled heart sounds, jugular venous distension, or hypotension, that would be consistent with pericardial tamponade.

D. There are no peritoneal signs or other acute physical findings to suggest bowel perforation and septic shock.

E. IV infiltration is a local reaction that occurs at the catheter site and would not explain these symptoms.

173. **B.** This patient's elevated anion and osmolal gap indicate that she may have ingested a toxic amount of alcohol in addition to the ethanol; therefore she requires supportive care while the levels are obtained.

A. This child has a very elevated ethanol level for her age and is not stable to go home. In addition, the metabolites of methanol, ethylene glycol, and isopropyl alcohol can be extremely toxic and dangerous. Fortunately, the coingestion of ethanol will result in the preferential inhibition of alcohol dehydrogenase, preventing metabolism of the toxic ethanols and acting as an antidote.

C. IV thiamine is important to replace with chronic alcoholism but would not be indicated in this patient.

D. Fomepizole is a potent inhibitor of alcohol dehydrogenase and can be used in the treatment of ethylene glycol or methanol ingestion. This is an expensive therapy that has not yet been widely used in children.

E. Hemodialysis is an effective and rapid technique to remove ethylene glycol and methanol and their toxic metabolites. Indications for hemodialysis would include severe metabolic acidosis, renal failure, or high levels of ethylene glycol or methanol.

174. **D.** The patient in this scenario is presenting with a retropharyngeal abscess. Classic symptoms include fever, dysphagia, neck swelling or pain, a muffled voice, drooling, or stridor. The lateral neck film reveals a widening of the retropharyngeal soft tissue (prevertebral) space as defined by more than one half of a vertebral body below C3. The diagnosis should be confirmed by CT scan to further evaluate the extent of the infection. Appropriate management consists of controlling the airway, use of parenteral antibiotics such as ampicillin-sulbactam, and drainage in a majority of patients.

A. Immediate consultation with anesthesia and intubation in the OR would be indicated if epiglottitis were suspected, unlikely in a case of a child with current vaccines and no evidence of stridor or respiratory distress. The classic x-ray finding is a swollen or thumbprint-like epiglottis.

B. The use of racemic epinephrine would be indicated in a scenario of croup.

C. Peritonsillar abscesses are more common in the adolescent population and rare in younger patients. The exam of the oropharynx should demonstrate unilateral tonsillar fullness with possible uvula deviation.

E. The use of dexamethasone would be indicated in cases where the abscess may cause upper airway inflammation significant enough to cause symptoms such stridor; it would also be indicated in the treatment of croup.

175. **D.** The clinical description of dry mucous membranes, cool extremities, prolonged capillary refill, doughy skin texture, and hypernatremia describes a child in hypovolemic shock. The treatment is intravascular volume expansion with isotonic fluid, such as 0.9% sodium chloride, 20 mL/kg per infusion, pushed IV followed by immediate reevaluation and repetition as needed to correct the clinical condition of shock.

A. Infusion of D5 (0.2%) NS plus 20 mEq/L at 1.5 maintenance may be appropriate after the initial phase of shock has been accomplished and the patient has been stabilized.

B. Infusion of 10 mL/kg of D10W is the treatment for hypoglycemia.

C. Administration of 2 mEq/kg sodium bicarbonate would be appropriate to correct a severe metabolic acidosis after the initial phase of fluid replacement has occurred.

E. Administration of IV antibiotics and an LP to rule out sepsis is not the initial management choice for a patient suffering from hypovolemic shock probably as a result of diarrhea.

176. **A.** D-Amphetamine is a sympathomimetic agent. Dilated pupils, diaphoresis, agitation, hyperthermia, and seizures would all be expected symptoms associated with toxicity from D-amphetamine or any other amphetamine-related product.

B. Agitation, rather than lethargy, would be an expected result of the ingestion of a sympathomimetic agent.

C. Diaphoresis, rather than dry skin, would be an expected side effect of D-amphetamine.

D. Hyponatremia would not be a likely result in this case.

E. GI symptoms may include nausea, vomiting, or diarrhea. Constipation would not be expected.

177. **D.** Cephalohematomas are a common occurrence in newborns. They do not cross suture lines of the skull, present as a fluctuant mass, and are the result of a subperiosteal hemorrhage. They can be rarely associated with skull fractures.

A. Subgaleal hemorrhages are rare conditions that must be diagnosed quickly, as a relatively large amount of blood can collect and shock can occur. They are often associated with vacuum deliveries.

B. Molding is a normal finding in newborns. Commonly it is seen after prolonged delivery.

C. Caput succedaneum is swelling that is noted after birth and crosses the suture lines.

E. Scalp monitoring is used for prolonged labor. As this baby was delivered quickly en route to the ED, there was no opportunity for scalp monitor placement.

178. **A.** Since the release of the Haemophilus vaccine, the incidence of epiglottitis due to this organism has dropped greatly. Other agents, such as *Streptococcus pyogenes, S. pneumoniae*, and *Staphylococcus aureus*, now represent a larger proportion of pediatric cases of epiglottitis.

B. Anxiety-provoking interventions should always be avoided in patients with epiglottitis. Phlebotomy, IV line placement, placing the child supine, or direct visualization of the oral cavity should be delayed until the airway is secure.

C. Patients with epiglottitis do not show the typical barky cough seen in viral croup. Stridor is a late finding and may not be present until the airway is nearly completely obstructed. Epiglottitis is a potentially lethal condition in which a child may develop air hunger, restlessness, cyanosis, and coma in just hours.

D. The classic finding on lateral neck radiographs is the "thumb sign" consistent with the large, swollen, cherry-red epiglottis seen on laryngoscopy. The "steeple" sign results from subglottic edema and is seen in viral croup, not epiglottitis.

E. Patients suspected of having epiglottitis should never be taken to the radiology department until after endotracheal intubation (or tracheostomy if necessary) is performed to prevent complete airway obstruction, regardless of the degree of respiratory distress.

179. **A.** This boy has the classic picture of DIC with widespread activation of the coagulation system, usually resulting from some form of shock, in this case septic shock.

B. There are no abnormalities of the PT or PTT in ITP.

C. Children with HUS present with renal insufficiency and a microangiopathic hemolytic anemia.

D. A Kasabach-Merritt phenomenon is associated with large hemangiomas that consume both platelets and clotting factors.

E. Elevated levels of D-dimer can be seen in deep venous thrombosis; however, microangiopathic changes of the red cells are rarely seen.

180. **D.** The patient in this scenario is presenting with pericarditis with impending cardiac tamponade. The chest x-ray shows evidence of an enlarged heart with increased pulmonary marking. Pulsus paradoxus is caused by the normal slight decrease in systolic arterial pressure during inspiration. With cardiac tamponade, this is exaggerated because of decreased filling of the left side of the heart. To hear the first Korotkoff sound, use a manometer while the patient takes a normal inspiration, and then listen to when the first Korotkoff sound is heard continuously. The difference between the two points is the pulsus paradoxus. If it is greater than 20 in a child with pericarditis, it is indicative of cardiac tamponade.

A, B, C. The impaired filling of the heart leads to distended jugular veins, narrow pulses, and a compensatory tachycardia.

E, F. An ECHO is the most sensitive technique for evaluating the pericardial effusion and looking for evidence of tamponade, but an ECG typically reveals widespread low-voltage QRS complexes with mild ST segment elevation and T wave inversion. Electrical alternans can be seen with a variable QRS complex amplitude.

181. **E.** Hemophilia A, hemophilia B, lupus anticoagulant, factor XI deficiency, and von Willebrand disease can all cause an isolated prolongation of the PTT. Von Willebrand disease is the most common inherited bleeding disorder, affecting 1% to 2% of the population. It is inherited in either an autosomal dominant or recessive manner. It typically presents with recurrent epistaxis or prolonged menstruation.

A, B. Factor VIII and IX deficiency are inherited in an X-linked pattern. Therefore, females are carriers and only extremely rarely affected.

C. Lupus anticoagulant is associated with thrombosis, not bleeding.

D. Factor XI deficiency is an autosomal recessive trait, though much more rare than von Willebrand disease.

182. **D.** The classic history of nighttime pain relieved by nonsteroidal anti-inflammatory drugs (NSAIDs), coupled with the radiographic findings of a sclerotic bone surrounding a radiolucent area, is consistent with the diagnosis of an osteoid osteoma. This is a benign bone tumor that may require resection if pain becomes intolerable.

A. Growing pains are worse at night and are relieved by NSAIDS, but they are typically bilateral and accompanied by a normal physical exam and normal radiographs.

B. There is no history of fever, limp, or systemic illness that would suggest osteomyelitis.

C. Although osteosarcomas are often diagnosed during adolescence and periods of rapid bone growth, the typical radiographic appearance is one of severely sclerotic bone with overlying new bone formation (Figure 182B).

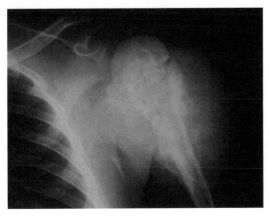

Figure 182B · Image courtesy of the Department of Radiology, Phoenix Children's Hospital, Phoenix, Arizona.

E. The classic radiograph findings of eosinophilic granuloma are more lytic, punched out-type lesions. Patients often present in early childhood and have systemic or skin involvement in a large proportion of cases.

183. **A.** Many would argue that follow-up is not even necessary for a single suspected vasovagal episode. Of all the options listed, discharge home and follow-up with cardiology for a 24-hour Holter monitor is the only option that is appropriate.

B. This patient clearly does not need ICU monitoring because the etiology is most likely a vasovagal syncope.

C. An ECHO would not be helpful in this scenario given the normal physical exam and past medical history.

D. An arterial line would be invasive and useless in a patient with a normal blood pressure.

E. Referral to psychology/psychiatry would only be appropriate if the patient was willfully fainting as can be seen following hyperventilation—something unlikely in this case.

184. **A.** Emesis occurring prior to 6 hours after ingestion implies significant iron ingestion. The absence of emesis 6 hours postingestion virtually excludes the diagnosis of iron poisoning.

B, D, E. Laboratory parameters and radiographs are not usually helpful with the exception of a confirmatory iron level. It is important to understand that iron poisoning is a clinical diagnosis and iron levels or other laboratory values do not dictate treatment.

C. Iron exerts its initial toxic effect on the gastric mucosa by direct irritation. Nausea, vomiting, and diarrhea may occur with accompanying electrolyte abnormalities. However, aside from the associated vomiting and diarrhea, a child may appear alert and playful without any other signs following iron ingestion.

185. **D.** The patient presents with signs of decompensated hypotensive shock after major trauma. He is tachycardic, hypotensive, and poorly perfused. Aggressive stabilization with attention to ensuring a stable airway, adequate oxygenation and ventilation, and improved circulation is mandatory. Of the answers provided, only repeat immediate volume expansion with an additional rapid infusion of 20 mL/kg isotonic crystalloid is immediately appropriate.

A. Although this patient will need to be admitted to the PICU, it is important to continue his initial resuscitation and attempt further stabilization of his circulation.

B. The possibility that the patient suffered a head injury following this accident needs to be considered, but further stabilization needs to occur before being sent for a CT scan.

C. Blunt abdominal trauma is common and an abdominal CT would be warranted after stabilization.

E. Placement of a femoral central line would be a useful form of IV access to supply more fluids but not simply to monitor or assess central venous pressure.

186. **D.** This patient has the clinical picture that is typical of a perforated acute appendicitis. Perforation is much more common in very young children. When perforation occurs, patients require IV fluid resuscitation and broad-spectrum antibiotics (ampicillin, gentamycin, clindamycin) for treatment of peritonitis for several hours prior to appendectomy. Antibiotics should provide coverage for *E. coli*, *Klebsiella*, *Pseudomonas*, and anaerobes. The patient should be placed on NG suction and be given nothing to eat or drink by mouth. Following the appendectomy, patients with perforation may develop paralytic ileus and bowel obstruction, persistent fever, abdominal abscess, wound infection, and/or sepsis.

A. Although this patient will eventually require surgical intervention, it is important to first stabilize the patient with particular attention to the ABCs (airway, breathing, circulation), while providing adequate antibiotic therapy to control the further progression of disease.

B. The patient has evidence of an acute surgical abdomen and should not be given anything by mouth.

C. As in the explanation for D, broad-spectrum antibiotics should be initiated to control the further progression of disease.

E. There is no need for a microscopic examination or culture of the stool in this case. Such tests may be valuable in suspected infectious gastroenteritis. In gastroenteritis, diarrhea is common and the vomiting and fever usually precede the abdominal pain.

187. **C.** Painless rectal bleeding in this age group without any signs of intestinal obstruction is most likely due to a Meckel diverticulum. Hemorrhage is the result of peptic ulceration and is typically bright red or maroon and painless. A Meckel scan uses technetium, which is excreted by the gastric mucosa and will demonstrate increased intake at the site of the diverticulum.

A. In this patient, a flat plate of the abdomen will typically show nonspecific findings.

B. Abdominal ultrasound is not specific for diagnosing Meckel diverticulum and is not the study of choice for GI bleeding.

D. CT of the abdomen may be helpful if the Meckel scan is normal and a colonoscopy does not reveal the source of the lower GI blood loss. It would not be the study of choice in a patient with GI bleeding unless there was a history of trauma or an abdominal mass.

E. An upper GI will not demonstrate a diverticulum near the level of the ileum.

188. **D.** The patient presented in the case scenario has typical findings of acute mastoiditis. Acute mastoiditis is caused by extension of infection from otitis media into the mastoid air cells. The presentation usually includes fever, ear pain, postauricular swelling and erythema, and a protruding pinna. The common causative organisms are *Streptococcus pneumoniae*, *Streptococcus pyogenes*, and *Staphylococcus aureus*. The initial treatment should combine IV, broad-spectrum antibiotic administration with drainage of the middle ear (myringotomy).

A. Oral amoxicillin does not provide adequate coverage for the common causative organisms.

B. While ceftriaxone may provide adequate antibiotic coverage, most patients should be hospitalized and observed for complications such as meningitis, sepsis, brain abscess, venous sinus thrombosis, osteomyelitis, labyrinthitis, or Bezold (deep neck) abscess.

C. Cefuroxime alone without drainage of the middle ear is not considered optimal treatment.

E. Mastoidectomy is usually reserved for cases in which antibiotics and drainage do not result in marked improvement in 48 hours.

---

189. **C.** Diphenhydramine (Benadryl) toxicity is associated with agitation, dry mouth, dry axilla, flushed skin, tachycardia, and hyperthermia due to its anticholinergic effects.

A. Acetaminophen toxicity is most likely to present with nausea, vomiting, abdominal pain, and anorexia, which may progress to jaundice and liver failure.

B. Propranolol ingestion is likely to produce bradycardia, hypotension, lightheadedness, fatigue, nausea, and vomiting.

D. Lithium overdosage may result in nausea, vomiting, tremor, drowsiness, and lack of muscle coordination.

E. Phenytoin may cause nystagmus, tremor, ataxia, and dysarthria. Severe overdose may result in respiratory and circulatory depression.

---

190. **C.** Unfortunately, the use of amphetamines and derivatives is quite common in the United States. Substances such as methamphetamine and MDMA are actually becoming more of a problem in recent years. While the above presentation could indeed be the result of these substances, it is important to complete a thorough examination with appropriate lab evaluation. The ABCs are the important priorities.

A. Often, street drugs have more than one active substance whether the buyer knows this or not. Lab analysis of the pills is important but often is a later source of information.

B. Ipecac is not appropriate in this setting as emesis can cause more problems in an altered level of consciousness. Activated charcoal is more likely to be of benefit in unknown ingestions.

D. It is necessary to proceed with the ABCs and provide supportive care rather than simple observation.

E. Further identification of the pills will not immediately help in the management of this patient.

---

191. **D.** Erythema of the TM alone is rarely indicative of acute otitis media. Normal eardrum position and normal mobility with pneumatic otoscopy should be interpreted as normal. Many babies without ear pathology pull at or play with their ears.

A. The most important diagnostic features of acute otitis media are a bulging TM, and decreased mobility when positive and negative pressure are applied into the ear canal with a rubber bulb attached to the otoscope (pneumatic otoscopy). There is often pain. Fever is present in only about 50% of cases, but almost all ear infections are preceded by URI symptoms.

B. Otitis media with effusion, previously known as serous otitis media, is caused by a blocked eustachian tube. The TM is usually in the retracted position secondary to a negative middle ear pressure. Fluid levels and air bubbles are often seen through the TM. Most patients do not have pain, but temporary conductive hearing loss is common.

C. The eardrum in bullous myringitis has hemorrhagic or serous bubble-like blisters on the TM. This condition is caused by the same organisms that cause acute otitis media. The patient usually has a great deal of ear pain.

E. When the eardrum perforates in acute otitis media, the ear canal generally becomes filled with purulent material and the TM is not visible. A more chronic perforation may appear as a dark hole in the TM. Pneumatic otoscopy will be abnormal with decreased or absent mobility.

192. **C.** The most appropriate next step would involve obtaining a complete blood count, blood culture, and plain radiographs of the foot.

A, B. Obtaining plain films before going straight to a bone scan or MRI is preferable. The suspected injury and inoculation occurred approximately 15 days ago. Radiographic findings of a fracture or osteomyelitis should be evident on plain films. If further suspicion is still high and plain radiographs are negative, an MRI or bone scan may then be indicated.

D. Simply applying a splint without first determining the extent of injury would be inappropriate.

E. Obtaining a blood culture before giving antibiotics is a good general principle.

193. **A.** Osteomyelitis causes soft tissue swelling around the infected bone and subperiosteal fluid collections and reaction. This diagnosis also makes sense given the mechanism and timing of the injury and physical findings.

B, C, D. Simple cellulitis, nail bed avulsion, or a right ankle sprain would not cause the bony changes seen on radiograph.

E. ALL should show a majority of lymphoblasts on the CBC and bony changes, if any, should be in the marrow. Occasionally leukemic infiltrates can present as destructive, sclerotic-type lesions seen on plain films.

194. **D.** Todd paralysis is temporary hemiparesis following a focal seizure and may be confused with a stroke. The symptoms should completely resolve within 24 hours of the seizure. Observation is likely warranted in the hospital given the weakness and risk of falling at home.

A, C. A cerebral angiogram and head MRI/MRA are used in the evaluation for stroke and are unnecessary in this case of Todd paralysis.

B. PICU admission is unnecessary if the patient is hemodynamically and neurologically stable; neurosurgical consultation is not indicated.

E. An LP and CSF analysis are not useful or necessary for cases of simple Todd paralysis.

195. **B.** Plain films of the chest and neck are indicated to look for radio-opaque foreign bodies and to assess for the presence of any hyperinflation of the involved hemithorax.

A. CT is too costly and may require sedation in a young child.

C, D. A modified barium swallow and upper GI series are used to assess for swallowing dysfunction and gastroesophageal reflux disease, not acute lung pathology.

E. Cervical spine x-rays are used to assess for bony injuries after trauma and are not indicated in this scenario.

196. **E.** This child's skull radiograph shows evidence of periventricular calcifications consistent with a possible diagnosis of congenital CMV. The child's developmental delay would also be consistent with the diagnosis. Congenital infection occurs in 1% of all newborns and may manifest itself in the immediate newborn period as sepsis with hepatosplenomegaly and growth retardation. Another 10% to 20% of infants may be asymptomatic at birth but progress to sequelae consisting of developmental delay, seizures, retinitis, and deafness. Although this child's work-up may be completed as an outpatient, the most appropriate choice listed is admission to the hospital.

A. Neurosurgical consultation is not indicated at this time.

B. A head CT would be useful in the continued management of this patient and probably would have been preferred over simple radiograph for better visualization of intracranial injury/hemorrhage following the fall; an MRI is not as useful in detecting calcifications.

C. There is no reason to suspect abuse in this patient; there is no delay in treatment nor is the injury inconsistent with the mother's story.

D. The child has developmental delay and periventricular calcifications that need further evaluation.

197. **A.** β-Blockers may lead to unopposed α blockade that may cause hypertension and worsening ischemia in the setting of cocaine abuse. In general, β-blockers are not indicated in toxin-induced tachycardia.

B, C. Although amphetamine and PCP abuse is expected to result in agitation and tachycardia, myocardial ischemia secondary to either of these drugs has not been definitively shown to be worsened with a β-blocker. However, as in the explanation for A, β-blockers are generally not indicated in toxin-induced tachycardia.

D, E. Heroin and codeine would not be expected to result in significant tachycardia. The expected toxic side effects would be bradycardia and respiratory depression.

198. **B.** Head CT is the most appropriate choice of imaging study.

A. According to the AAP practice guideline, *The Management of Minor Closed Head Injury in Children*, a skull radiograph is not sensitive enough to pick up intracranial injuries. (Committee on Quality Improvement, American Academy of Pediatrics, Commission on Clinical Policies and Research, and American Academy of Family Physicians. The management of minor closed head injury in children. Pediatrics 1999;104:1407–1415.)

C. Head MRI has no added benefit than head CT and costs more.

D. Bone scans would not show intracranial injuries.

E. Head ultrasounds are not sensitive enough to detect skull fractures.

199. **C. Given the baby's drowsiness and poor feeding, in-hospital observation is warranted.**

A, B. Home observation would be risky, even with a responsible adult.

D. Neurosurgical consultation is warranted with depressed skull fractures, but not generally for a simple, nondepressed fracture without any intracranial injury.

E. Rapid sequence intubation and hyperventilation are used in the intensive care setting for severe head injuries showing signs of increased intracranial pressure.

200. **D. Depressed skull fractures must be treated surgically if a neurologic deficit is present, if a compound wound is present, or if the depression is greater than 3 to 5 mm.**

A, B. Given the new diagnosis, home observation would be wholly inappropriate, even with a responsible adult.

C. Simple admission to the hospital for observation without neurosurgical involvement is not appropriate.

E. Rapid sequence intubation and hyperventilation are used in the intensive care setting for severe head injuries showing signs of increased intracranial pressure. In this case, the child has no obvious intracranial injuries or clinical exam that would necessitate intubation at this time.

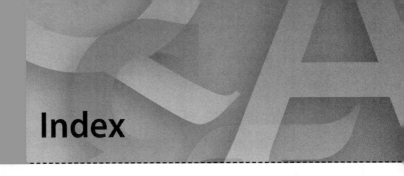

Index

Index note: page references with an *f* or a *t* indicate a figure or table on designated page; page references in **bold** indicate discussion of the subject in the Answers and Explanations sections.